MY PATIENT – MY NURSE

MY PATIENT – MY NURSE

A Guide to Primary Nursing

Stephen G Wright
RGN, DipN, RCNT, DANS, RNT, MSc

Consultant Nurse, Nursing Development Unit
(Care of the Elderly), Tameside General Hospital

with contributors

SCUTARI PRESS
London

A division of Scutari Projects, the publishing company of the Royal College of Nursing

First published 1990
Reprinted 1992
Reprinted 1993

British Library Cataloguing in Publication Data

Wright, Stephen G.
  My patient—my nurse.
  1. Medicine. Nursing
  I. Title
  610.73

  ISBN 1-871364-32-9

Typeset, printed and bound by The Alden Press, Osney Mead, Oxford

Contents

To
the staff and patients
of the
Nursing Development Unit

Contributors

I am grateful to all my colleagues for the comments and help given in the writing of this text. It was through our experiences and discussions of primary nursing that the idea for the book originated.

Apart from contributing in a general sense to the examples throughout this text, each of my colleagues from the Nursing Development Unit (NDU) provided detailed work to enable me to write certain specific sections:

Susan Archer, RGN, RM, (formerly Night Sister and currently Ward Sister/Senior Primary Nurse in the NDU) on the role of night staff (Chapter 3);

Philip Gartside, RGN, (Charge Nurse and Senior Primary Nurse in the NDU) on the various roles in primary nursing (Chapters 3 and 4);

Nasrin Khadim, RGN, FETC, (formerly Ward Sister in the NDU and currently Clinical Nurse Specialist) on the setting up of primary nursing and the involvement of the teacher (Chapters 4 and 5);

Elsie Purdy, RGN, (Senior Nurse Manager in the NDU) on the role of the nurse manager (Chapter 5);

Gillian Wills, RGN, SEN, FETC, (Primary Nurse in the NDU) on organisational matters and evaluation (Chapters 4 and 6).

Foreword

'Primary nursing is more than a simple way of organising nurses; it is a voyage into nursing's little-explored territories, a journey into a new reality.' So claim Steve Wright and his colleagues in this splendidly readable book. And they invite their readers to enter, with them, into the world of primary nursing. In so doing, they show how the vision of primary nursing transforms the understanding of the nature of nursing and also how primary nursing can be achieved in very practical ways.

The essence of primary nursing is encapsulated in the concepts of fellowship and companionship. Its purpose is to enable each patient to relate to 'my nurse' and each nurse to develop a special relationship with 'my patient'. Nurse and patient accompany each other during the patient's voyage through illness, dependency, recovery – or the valley of the shadow of death. The opportunity that primary nursing provides for nurses and patients to develop this deep companionship is a vital factor in the healing potential inherent in nursing.

Steve Wright and his colleagues move on from a convincing general discussion of the value of primary nursing to a detailed and equally convincing discussion of practicalities. They provide answers to some of the most worrying 'Twenty Questions' that confront nurses who might want to adopt primary nursing. In so doing, they share some of the problems they have experienced and the solutions they have found, with regard to issues such as the role of the ward sister/charge nurse, the contribution of enrolled nurses, night duty and access to nursing notes.

The authors finish with the challenge 'Pursue your

vision!' Having read this book, and seen this vision in practice in their unit, I hope that many nurses will rise to the challenge, share the vision and achieve the reality, for their own benefit and, ultimately all-important, for the benefit of their patients.

Caroline Cox, BSc(Soc), MSc(Econ), RGN, FRCN

Preface

The Nursing Development Unit in the Care of the Elderly Unit at Tameside General Hospital was formally set up in 1986. It was the culmination of many years of previous work, aimed at producing change in nursing practice for the older patient. From the start, it was one of our goals to implement primary nursing – not just as a means of organising care, but as part of the whole way in which we think about nursing, and how it should be practised.

Since those early days, almost 10 years ago, we have witnessed the entry of primary nursing into the debating forum of nursing and its growth in many sections of health care. Many nurses have visited the unit to find out about primary nursing, or have quizzed our staff at various courses and conferences as to how it might be done.

Inevitably, the concerns and questions of many nurses proved to be the same: How many staff do you need? What about the doctors? Can the enrolled nurse be a primary nurse? What can the manager do? and so on, and so on.

This book is in part a response to those uncertainties. We have tried to produce very much a 'how to do it' text that will answer many of those questions and deal with the practicalities of primary nursing in the everyday world of the nurse. At the same time, we hope to share with the reader a vision of what primary nursing might be, which is more than a mere system to deploy nurses differently. Aiming for the goal of primary nursing brings with it a wholesale reappraisal of what nursing is and how nurses should work with each other, their patients, colleagues, visitors and other carers.

We have tried to fill this book with our own experiences and views, and, in so doing, we hope that you, the reader, whether doubtful or enthusiastic, will enhance your own knowledge of primary nursing. Perhaps if you are just beginning the journey towards primary nursing, you will find it less fraught with difficulties, avoid some of the pitfalls and reach your destination sooner if you are armed with the knowledge of how others have travelled the path before. It is our experience and our belief that primary nursing can help nurses do their job better, with benefit to both patients and themselves, and this, after all, is what matters.

Throughout the text the word 'patient' is used for simplicity. 'Client', 'resident', or any other word the reader is familiar with for the recipient of care, is equally applicable.

Steve Wright and colleagues
December 1988

Acknowledgements

The authors would like to thank the following for their help:

Mr R Butterworth, Unit General Manager, and Mr M L Johnson, Assistant Unit General Manager, for their continuing support in enabling it all to happen and for their kind permission to reproduce the job descriptions in the Appendix.

Mr R Davenport, Unit General Manager when the Nursing Development Unit was created, Mr W A Bamber, also a former Unit General Manager, and the senior medical staff, Dr M A Matin, Dr A H Wan, Dr O M P Jolobe and Dr Sil, for their encouragement of nursing.

Mr T W Fisher, OBE, Assistant General Manager (Quality Assurance) and Chief Nurse Adviser, for his interest and support.

Mary Underwood, Care Assistant in the Nursing Development Unit, for her permission to include an extract from her 1989 project on primary nursing in Chapter 3.

Special thanks must also go to Mrs Irene Hill for assistance above and beyond the call of duty, and to Mr Ian Webster and Mrs M McDermott for their invaluable help and many cups of tea.

The Tameside Nursing Development Unit image and logo were designed by Total Concept Design (UK) Ltd, Manchester.

CHAPTER 1

The Essence of
Primary Nursing

Fellowship is heaven, and lack of fellowship is hell;
fellowship is life, and the lack of fellowship death;
and the deeds that ye do upon the earth, it is for
fellowship's sake that ye do them.

William Morris
The Dream of John Ball

Traditional views of the history of nursing tend to follow a
very typical model. Nursing is seen as constantly progress-
ing, marching forward in time, while forever improving,
overcoming great odds and striving towards excellence.

A closer examination of the past might raise a few
questions over this view. Whole forests must have been
felled to produce the paper for a veritable mountain of
reports, research documents and royal commissions. They
span many decades and indicate that in fact all is not well
with nursing, nor has it been for some time. There are many
deep-rooted problems in nursing; much does not appear to
have changed fundamentally over the years.

Two principal perspectives seem to emerge – those of the
patient and of the nurse.

The Patient's View

Much recent work (e.g. Henderson, 1980; Lanara, 1981; Health Service Ombudsman, 1986; Pearson, 1988a, b) illustrates a continued dissatisfaction of patients with the quality of care which they receive, particularly concerning the quality of the nurse–patient relationship. The Health Service Ombudsman's reports (1986, 1987, 1988), for example, indicate dissatisfaction with nursing, which has many common threads – failures in communication, uncaring attitudes, inattention to needs – quite apart from failings in expertise associated with many physical tasks such as attention to hygiene or wound care. Pearson (1988a, b) has noted how 'patients themselves agree with the view that nurses are obsessed with the performance of tasks associated with physical care and the support of medical regimes, and that they do not fulfil expectations as the humanisers of the health care systems'. Patients appear to· want a positive, healing, helpful relationship with nurses, yet so often nurses are told not to 'get involved' with patients. Nursing, on the contrary, is about being 'involved' with patients, but it is an involvement within defined limits that they seek, a therapeutic relationship for the patient that does not harm him while at the same time does not damage or exhaust the nurse. Primary nursing is about the redefining of that relationship and the role of the nurse in it. The primary nurse is nothing if not 'involved' with the patient.

The challenge of primary nursing is to overcome these weaknesses. This is not, however, to suggest that nurses should 'throw the baby out with the bathwater'! Nursing has many valuable qualities and these should be cherished and built upon. The call to primary nursing is not to suggest that everything before has been bad – it has not – and that, if we would but implement primary nursing, everything in the future would be perfect – it would not. Rather it is a call to look more closely at what nurses and patients value and to redefine how nurses should think and act in the light of these needs.

Lanara (1981) argues that 'nursing today is at a critical

and, one might say, tragic crossroads. The nurse is better educated, more knowledgeable and more science-orientated. Yet the patient, for all the superb physical and technical improvements in his environment, feels lonely and even abandoned, because nobody cares for him as a person'. Lanara goes on to suggest that for nurses the way forward is to re-examine and define their beliefs, enriching what already exists, to bring about 'the awakening of the spirit of nursing, which, integrated with science and technology, will re-create the living spirit in a matrix of concern'.

Some years ago, I was involved in a survey of patients' and staff opinions on what constituted 'good' nursing (Wright, 1987a). This preliminary work aimed at devising some quality assurance tools. In the survey, nurses tended to see the 'good' nurse as being 'hard working', 'tidy', 'efficient', 'carrying out procedures correctly', and so on.

Interestingly, many of the patients seemed to lay more emphasis on different issues. One patient summed this up quite succinctly. 'Look, it's like this, when I come into your ward, I want to feel the nurse *cares* for me. I'd rather she told me what's going on than keep washing me all the time. When I come through the doors of your ward, I want a nurse who says: "Hello, I'm Nurse so-and-so, I've been expecting you. I'm going to look after you while you're here. If you want to know anything, I'll keep you informed, and your wife too! So first I'll settle you in bed. After that, we'll spend some time together sorting out what we can do to help so you know where you're going"'.

This particular patient went on to describe in graphic detail what the qualities of 'his' nurse should be – informing, teaching, supporting, being 'on his side', involving his family, keeping him safe, and so on. The extraordinary common sense of this patient made me look again at how I and my colleagues projected ourselves, and gave new impetus to our innovations on making care more personal.

Consultant nurse

THE NURSE'S VIEW

If patients are not always fully satisfied with nursing, then there is also parallel dissatisfaction among nurses. Nurses demonstrate this with their feet, producing an attrition rate so great that nursing must reproduce itself every 10 years simply to keep enough nurses at the bedside (RCN, 1986). Other documents mirror the American experience of the 'Magnet Hospitals' study (McLure et al, 1983), indicating that, while nurses' salary levels contribute to the exodus, equally important are high levels of dissatisfaction with the 'climate' (created by negative management attitudes) in which they work, and the sense of powerlessness at being unable to practise nursing in the manner in which they feel they should (Dean, 1988; Price Waterhouse, 1988; Strong and Robinson, 1988).

Primary nursing suggests that nurses should practise with greater professional autonomy. It also opens the way for nurses to achieve job satisfaction by extending their relationship with the patient, so that they know they are meeting his needs. Thus, while primary nursing can do little to address itself to nurses' pay, it has the potential to deal with those other dissatisfactions in nurses related to the organisation of care.

PRIMARY NURSING – A HISTORICAL BACKGROUND

To some extent, primary nursing is a return to what Nightingale (1869) defined as her 'case method' approach to nursing – an individual (trained) nurse being responsible for a given group of patients, dealing with a variety of issues related to health, hygiene and family support. While the education (and hence knowledge base) of the Nightingale nurses was not as highly developed as in more recent times (nor was the notion of the 'professional nurse'), there are many commonalities. To that extent, primary nursing might be seen as a return to the case method, a rediscovery perhaps of what is at the heart of nursing.

The post-Nightingale era witnessed a growing hospital base for nursing and the rise of the scientific medical model dominating health care. Shortages of nurses (especially during war time) compounded the problem. The result was the evolution of the 'task-centred' approach to care. Lee (1979) notes how task-centred nursing follows an industrial model, breaking down care into groups of (nursing) tasks carried out by nurses according to skill and status (the 'back round', the 'obs round', the 'toilet round'). Beyers and Philips (1971) note that the 'case method' was 'expensive in terms of professional nursing salaries and impractical for most nursing units'. In part, argues Menzies (1961), the tasks also became a means of containing anxiety. Unable to cope with the difficulties of working in large bureaucratic organisations and with the stress of dealing with the totality of the patient and his problems, nurses responded, Menzies argues, by dividing aspects of the patients' care into neat chunks which could be more easily managed. Henderson (1980) suggests that this ultimately proved satisfying to neither patient nor nurse. Both were dehumanised in the process: completing the tasks does not remove the sense of failure on the part of the nurse from seeing how much care has *not* been given, while the patient is short-changed on care which cannot easily be task allocated (e.g. teaching or comforting).

Efforts to break away from the reductionist industrialised approach inherent in task-centred nursing led to developments in team nursing (Waters, 1985) and patient allocation (Marks-Maran, 1978). However, these methods (while seeming to have fewer nurses caring for fewer patients, for large periods of time, and hence making care more personal) are open to abuse. Nurses working in teams still tend to split care into tasks amongst the team. Patient allocation leaves open the question of the level of expertise of the nurse to whom the patient is allocated (auxiliary? student? trained nurse?) and the length of time of the allocation. Furthermore, accountability and autonomy in both these methods remain unclear.

> We'd organised the ward for a long time on the basis of patient allocation. For us, moving to primary nursing was the next logical step. In that sense, we found that patient allocation was the precursor of primary nursing.
>
> *Ward sister/primary nurse*

To some degree, therefore, the advent of primary nursing

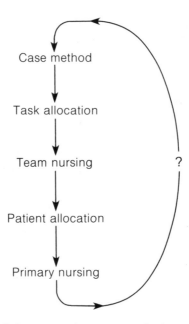

Fig. 1.1   Primary nursing as an evolutionary process

may be seen as an evolutionary process (Figure 1.1) with elements of a desire to return to certain earlier values and methods in the organisation of nursing care.

However, it would be a mistake to view these trends as a neat cycle of historical events. The birth of one has not necessarily led to the extinction of the other. All these methods of organising nursing can be found in practice simultaneously in many parts of nursing at present.

It is interesting to note also that the use of primary nursing as a dominant theme in recent years has occurred alongside two other major topics in nursing practice – the nursing process and nursing models. A full explanation of these last two issues is beyond the scope of this text, but it might be useful to examine briefly how they are linked to primary nursing (Figure 1.2).

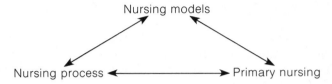

Fig. 1.2   The link between the nursing process, models and primary nursing

NURSING MODELS

Every nurse carries in his or her head an 'image' (Reilly, 1975) of what nursing is. This informal model, the way each nurse thinks about nursing, has important implications, for it determines the way in which the nurse acts out nursing. For example, the nurse's beliefs about the elderly, whether as hopeless cases or as individuals with potential for rehabilitation, will affect the way in which the nurse works with those patients. When nurses start to pool these beliefs, ideas and concepts about what nursing is, they can construct more formal models (Wright, 1986). The next step is then to decide how these are put into practice. If, for example, the notion that care should be 'individualised' is espoused, then how is it done? What is the best method of organisation to make care so personal: patient allocation? task allocation? primary nursing?

NURSING PROCESS

In carrying out nursing, another question arises. How does the nurse decide what help is needed? The nursing process might simply be described as the tool by which nursing is thought through. Thus, by assessing the patient for his needs, deciding what needs to be done (planning) and actually getting on with it (implementing), while at the same time making sure it is effective (evaluation), the 'process cycle' is established.

PRIMARY NURSING

This can therefore be seen as one option for nurses to put their beliefs and ideas about nursing into action, using the nursing process as a basis for working out the patient's care. Models, process and primary nursing are therefore all intimately linked (Figure 1.2), and it is the practice upon which the contributors to this book have based their work.

PRIMARY NURSING AS A CROSS-CULTURAL PROCESS

While many of the earlier writings on primary nursing (Hall, 1969; Manthey, 1970, 1973) have their origins in the USA, it should be emphasised that developments in primary nursing have taken place across the world. In that sense, it should be seen not as an import from one nation, but rather as a concurrent transcultural process. Descriptions and evaluations of primary nursing have emerged, for example, from:

- Australia (Watson, 1978)
- Japan (Otoya, 1979)
- UK (Lee, 1979; Sparrow, 1986)
- Norway (Aschjem et al, 1979)
- Belgium (Blanpain, 1976)
- The Netherlands (Van Eindhoven, 1979)
- Canada (Medaglia, 1978)

Manthey (1970) appears to have been the progenitor of the term 'primary nursing', but, in doing so, she seems to have focused on an idea with international implications. Nurses across the globe seem to share common concerns, goals and hopes in their desire to reaffirm nursing as a patient-centred practice. Primary nursing taps that transcultural nursing desire.

PRIMARY NURSING DEFINED

While patient allocation and the case method, for example, have in some ways offered directions for more personal care, they do not address themselves sufficiently to the principles of professional practice, accountability or the degrees of knowledge and skill which underpin them. Indeed, Hall (1969) derides team or task nursing as 'getting through the work' and the mark of a 'trade', not a profession, and thus a disservice to the patient. Patient allocation may be applied, for example, on an ad hoc basis and any grade of nurse might be used (Wright, 1987b), while the older case method relied upon the limited vision of the nurse's role available at the time (a weaker knowledge base and subservience to medical practice).

As Hegyvary (1982) notes, primary nursing 'is both a philosophy of care and an organisational design. It is not simply a way of assigning nurses to patients, but rather a view of nursing as a professional, patient-centred practice'. Manthey (1980) writes of the development of the 'my nurse' concept and provides one of the best definitions of primary nursing: 'The nursing care of a specific patient is under the continuous guidance of one nurse from admission through to discharge. One nurse on each shift provides total care for the same group of patients day after day. Round the clock care is co-ordinated for each patient by the nurse designated as the primary nurse for that patient'. The implications of putting into practice the above statement are profound, not only for the professionalisation of nursing and the effects on the quality of patient care, but also for the wider organisations and society in which the nurse works.

While Hall (1969) has dismissed non-primary nursing as having the characteristics of a 'trade', Manthey (1980) has referred to other forms as an attempt to 'deprofessionalise' nursing. Breaking down nursing into simple components, it is argued, emphasises a bureaucratic organisation of nursing, which does little to enhance the status of, and the satisfaction with, nursing, of both nurses and patients.

Rotkontch (1979) has argued that the term 'primary nursing' should not be used because of possible confusion with primary care. She regards the term 'professional nursing practice' as adequate. Hegyvary notes that these terms can become confusing because of over-use and misuse. Primary nursing, however, must be seen as a distinct entity.

A nurse in the community as part of a primary care team (i.e. promoting health outside the hospital setting) may be practising in either a task-centred or primary nursing way. 'Nursing is a profession only to the extent to which nursing performs professional roles; merely performing tasks or delegating everything to others does not meet the criteria [for professional nursing] . . . nor does holding the title "professional nurse" ensure that the nurse performs at a professional level' (Hegyvary, 1982). The issue of nursing as a profession is debatable, but primary nursing offers a professional model (see Chapter 6) which nurses can follow because it contains the following basic ingredients for professional practice:

- *Accountability.* The primary nurse is answerable for the nursing care of the patient or family 24 hours a day, while he is in her care in hospital or community.
- *Autonomy.* In the mode of 'professional self-governance', the primary nurse has the authority, and acts on it, to make decisions about the patient's, or family's, nursing care.
- *Co-ordination.* A smooth flow of nursing care exists from shift to shift with direct communication from caregiver to care-giver.
- *Comprehensiveness.* Each care-giver gives all the nursing care required during the course of a shift (sometimes called 'total patient care').

Primary nursing is essentially the function of the 'primary (registered) nurse'. In her absence, 'associate' nurses take over the nursing care, but they remain responsible to the primary nurse for carrying out the agreed plan of care or revising it as conditions change.

It is acknowledged (Manthey, 1980) that the above four elements are not always achievable absolutely in every situation, but it is argued that they 'set the standards or goals for defining the essence of primary nursing'. She notes how much depends on the abilities of the nurse and the nature of the organisational structure to achieve success. She comments: 'Primary nursing does not define or guarantee the quality of nursing care. As a system, it *facilitates* a very high level of quality by enabling and empowering individuals to perform at their maximum capacity' (Manthey, 1980). Thus, to modify Nightingale's (1869) earlier words defining nursing ('putting the patient in the best position for nature to act'), primary nursing puts the nurses in the best position for nursing to act.

Primary nursing is a challenge to nurses. It opens a 'can of worms', letting loose many aspects of nursing that they have chosen to hide from or ignore. Not every nurse will wish to be, or can be, a primary nurse, and perhaps many would wish to retreat when faced with the enormity of the implications. How far can the nurse be accountable? What will the nature of the relationship with the patients be, and how can it be managed? What sort of education or management is needed to foster primary nursing? How can it be organised? How will relationships with colleagues be affected? Who will be the primary nurse?

Primary nursing is a call to nurses to come out of their shells, to assert themselves and to seek answers to questions like these. The following chapters of this book will address themselves to these issues – and more.

Primary nursing means change, and, faced with the seeming enormity of the task, it is little wonder that many nurses might resist and retreat. Perhaps, after all, it would be better to keep things as they are and cloak the potential of nursing in the mantle of others (let the doctor or the sister tell me what to do!). As Kafka (1916) succinctly points out, 'sometimes it is safer to be in chains than to be free'. Primary nursing is more than a simple way of organising nurses; it is a voyage into nursing's little-explored territories, a journey into a new reality.

CHAPTER 2

Changing to Primary Nursing

Hos successus alit possunt
quia posse videntur

Success nourished them; they seemed
to be able, and so they were able

Virgil
The Aeneid

To develop primary nursing implies, inevitably, that things must change. If primary nursing is different from the status quo, there will be movement away from something (the way we always did things) towards something (our new way of doing things). Very often in nursing there has been a tendency to implement change by forcing it through, using a 'top-down' power–coercive approach, i.e. orders passed down through the hierarchy. Such an approach is fatally flawed, for staff forced into change will usually invent all manner of ways to resist, distort or disrupt the change. This happened in many parts of the UK with the implementation of the nursing process.

Another strategy is to use the 'hero-innovator' model (Georgiades and Phillimore, 1975), tapping the skills of a particular energetic and charismatic leader who attempts to lead the staff into change, only to burn out, leaving the change to collapse and return to the old order when she has gone (and, in so doing, proves the doubters right that the change would never work anyway!). It is equally difficult to implement change when impetus comes from only one or two staff in a particular setting, or when the enthusiast does not have the power and control to change things.

> I was really sold on primary nursing as soon as I read about it, and the conference just filled me with more enthusiasm. But where do I start? – I'm only the enrolled nurse. The charge nurse isn't going to listen to me, and the manager doesn't like anything that rocks the boat.
>
> After a while, I got the impression that I was on my own in this. I began to feel that people were leaving the clinic early to go on their rounds just to avoid talking to me about the subject.
>
> *Enrolled nurse (community)*

The theory and application of change are complex subjects, which it is beyond the scope of this text to explore in full. British texts are now emerging (Pearson, 1985; Wright, 1989) that suggest ways in which nurses at clinical level can change practice. Some of the salient points can be brought together to form a change strategy to help to ease the path through the change process.

A CHANGE STRATEGY

The move towards primary nursing needs to go hand in hand with a change strategy – planning the change as much as possible to minimise conflicts and promote progress and co-operation.

Salvage (1988) comments that 'shock, withdrawal and apathy' are among the responses that managers and colleagues can feel when the nurse 'breezes in with her bright new idea. To what extent are they inevitable aspects of human behaviour and to what extent can they be anticipated and outwitted?' It seems that part of the solution is to plan the change. This is supported by Pearson and Vaughan (1986), who contend that 'some changes occur because of things around us, but most changes cannot effectively occur without being planned. Planned change is inevitably easier to manage than change which is imposed, haphazard or misunderstood!'

Thus a nursing process type of problem-solving approach can be helpful as part of an overall strategy. This involves identifying all the various facets of a situation and working out how to overcome them (assessing and planning). For example: Are there key people who need to be convinced? What information is needed? What resources are required? and so on. Then a gradual implementation of the plan takes place, with careful monitoring and evaluation to determine how it is working. In practice, however, the change process is rarely so linear, and a successful change programme requires an immense amount of flexibility to take into account numerous other factors.

Turrill (1985) suggests that some of these other factors in the plan should include the following:

- *Getting people together to agree the core purpose of the organisation*: e.g. does primary nursing fit in with the goals of the ward or unit to make care individualised?
- *Sharing a vision of a better future.* Primary nursing requires its advocates to have that vision, knowing that it cannot be achieved overnight, but seeing the goal always on the horizon and working towards it. Lasting change will not occur unless a critical core of the staff in a given setting shares the same vision and is willing to work towards it.

> Most of the staff were doubtful or downright difficult, but it only took the few of us. Just three of us out of the whole ward shared the same wishes, but we persisted. We learnt, we worked at it, eventually we won through.
>
> *Primary nurse*

- *Setting the working principles.* Thus, in the case of primary nursing, the ground rules need to be laid, perhaps identifying clearly who does what within the team, where each member's responsibilities lie, and reaching agreements on how conflicts will be dealt with.

- *Mapping the environment*: identifying the implications for other individuals and groups, and how these might be dealt with, e.g. how will the doctors be approached on this? What do the other disciplines, relatives, patients and colleagues need to know? This includes working out in advance how to respond to them.
- *Transition management*: managing the problems that occur between the start and finish lines of the change. The task that each is required to do can be clearly spelled out, as well as what resources are needed, e.g. new forms of nursing documentation.
- *Resistance reduction*. Copious two-way communication is necessary so that the team have a chance to explain and explore their feelings, question, clarify and seek information. Involving other groups in the change, listening to their point of view and engaging their support help to reduce resistance.

> Because we were working more flexibly, we had some problems with the portering staff. They were getting angry because we were disrupting their schedule for collecting the meal trolleys. We invited them to some of the ward meetings and introduced them to patients who said how much better things were. When they (the porters) felt part of it, when they saw what we were doing was helping patients, they understood and looked at their own way of doing things so that they could help us.
>
> *Senior primary nurse/charge nurse*

- *Seeking commitment*. Identifying key groups and individuals and devising non-threatening ways of winning them over helps to draw them into the change process.

> It was really the nursing officer who was pushing for it. She thought primary nursing was a great idea, but we weren't so sure. We were impressed, though, when she joined us on the ward and worked as part of the team, showing us not only how it could be done but that it was possible, drawing more of us into it. She was there as our example, ready with the facts and the support.
>
> *Associate nurse*

Changing anything in nursing is no doubt easier if there is a culture of innovation. If the setting has a climate that encourages change and sees it as part of normal day-to-day work, change is very much easier. Much of the responsibility for this lies in the hands of the nurse manager, and this will be dealt with later in Chapter 5.

Other dimensions of a change strategy are explained by Ottoway (1976, 1980) and have been developed to apply to nursing settings (Pearson, 1985; Wright, 1989). Some of the main points (Figure 2.1) include the following:

- *The presence of a change agent.* A change agent is a key person knowledgeable in the subject and in how to change things. It is better if the change agent works on site, with the staff, involved in their day-to-day practice. The position in the hierarchy is also important, i.e. changing practice on a particular unit is easier if the

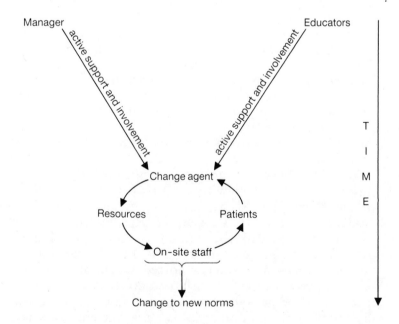

Fig. 2.1 Change strategy

designated change agent has more control (e.g. ward sister or charge nurse as opposed to enrolled nurse) in the organisation. Where nursing practice is changing, it is particularly helpful if the change agent has the credibility of being a practising nurse working with the staff. Managers and teachers who stand outside the organisation will find that getting staff to accept change will be more difficult.

- *Managers and educators*, where they are part of the clinical team, have a crucial part to play in giving support and guidance, staff counselling, supplying information and resources. If support of either of these groups is lacking, the change process will be hindered that much more.
- The *on-site staff* must be involved in the change process, whatever their status or role. For the change to be effective and long lasting, the new norms must be 'owned' by the staff. Ownership, through involvement in the decision-making process, taking account of views and using suggestions, is essential for new behaviours to be implemented. This 'bottom-up' approach ensures staff participation and the generation of change at clinical level. The change agent's role and skills here are very important in guiding and encouraging this process, without seeming to dominate and control. Otherwise the staff will perceive it as a 'top-down' process, merely responding to orders. There is then a risk, if the change agent leaves or is absent, that the on-site staff will revert to the old norms.
- *Resources*. These include the provision of equipment and information and reviewing the number and skill mix of the staff (see 'The Manager's Role' in Chapter 5). If the staff are not adequately resourced to pursue the changes, they may suffer guilt through failure, reject the changes or exhaust themselves in an effort to keep the changes going. Nurses are often exhorted to change, yet not always given the wherewithal to do it. It is futile, for example, to embark upon primary nursing unless there is a concurrent commitment to examine, and change where necessary, the number and mix of staff.

> I was told I could get on with primary nursing provided I made do with what I'd got. I didn't want more staff, just a review of the existing workforce. There are only three trained staff in this ward. The rest are auxiliaries. It's no use telling me I can change things, and then do nothing to help me do it.
>
> *Ward sister*

- *Patients*. If primary nursing is deemed to help patients, then they can and must be involved in the change towards it. More details of how this can be done appear in Chapter 4.
- *Time*. Dealing with the problems that arise, preparing the ground and seeing these changes through can take a long time. Often it is the preparatory work that takes the longest.

> We've had many visitors come to the unit to learn about primary nursing. Some of them, I felt, assumed they could pick up a few facts and implement it the next day. Hopefully, by the time we had related our experiences and gone through all the implications, they've been a little more realistic. I hope we haven't put them off, but enthusiasm needs to be tempered with practicality. Here, it took us the best part of 4 years before we really made headway. In that time, we had to attend to a lot of things to make care more personal, and we had to work with the managers to look at the mix of staff and change it. Originally about 80% of the workforce were nursing auxiliaries. You can't do primary nursing with that. Now, on average, it's been revised to about 65% trained staff. The whole place had to change. It was wheels within wheels, because we couldn't have recruited the trained staff unless we'd done something about the image of the care of the elderly to attract the staff in the first place. We had to work towards primary nursing, passing through patient allocation first. Some people say primary nursing is easier in the care of the elderly – they should try it! Every place has its difficulties; they are just different difficulties in different places.
>
> *Consultant nurse*

Thus it can take many years for the groundwork to be done so that a setting becomes 'ripe' for primary nursing. This 'ripeness' is characterised by the shared values of the staff and the readiness to change. However, every setting will be different, and some may have the initial foundations which allow for a very rapid transition. Once there is a general readiness for primary nursing, then the ward or unit is at the 'get set' point. The next stage is the actual implementation, which on average seems to take about 18 months (this is a view derived from the experience of the contributors). For some it may be faster, for others, slower, depending upon the many variables:

Phase I The groundwork – perhaps years!

Phase II 6 months – preparing the staff. Reading about primary nursing; attending lectures; having meetings; planning the changes and how they will be managed; discussing primary nursing with others more experienced.

Phase III 6 months – the trial period. Putting the plans into action, all the time reviewing them; talking to each other; trying out the practice; identifying problems and overcoming them.

Phase IV 6 months of consolidation, rethinking and replanning. Refining the organisation of primary nursing and planning the moves towards perfection and identifying the limitations.

Planning the time phase, and making it realistic, is essential. Hoping for too much too soon can lead the staff to become dismayed and disillusioned. For example, leaping from task-centred care to primary nursing can be difficult for some; perhaps a transition phase, working at patient allocation first, can be helpful.

- *The choice of site.* It has been suggested that there is a time when a nursing unit becomes 'ripe' for primary nursing. This is rather difficult to define, but seems to be a combination of staff readiness, appropriate skill mix, staff willingness to try it, the supportive management climate and the knowledge and enthusiasm in sufficient key staff. Changing practice does not require everyone to be an enthusiastic innovator, but a small percentage of the workforce is sufficient to begin this transition. Some will lead, others will follow.

It seems that choosing the site, e.g. a ward or a team of community nurses where there is a willingness to learn and experiment, to act as a pilot scheme, is helpful. Other staff in other areas can learn from these schemes and perhaps reduce their own difficulties when they can learn from the experience of others. When one site is successful, then, rather like a germ, the idea can spread gradually from place to place, as Figure 2.2 illustrates.

This chapter has explained the concept of change in relation to primary nursing. There is no doubt that, as Machiavelli (1514) observed:

'There is nothing more difficult to handle, more doubtful of success, and more dangerous to carry through, than initiating

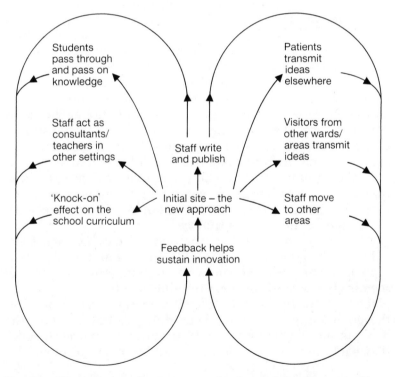

Fig. 2.2 Transmission of primary nursing beyond the pilot site. (From Wright, 1986. Reproduced by kind permission of Edward Arnold)

changes in a state constitution. The innovator makes enemies of all those who progressed under the old order, and only lukewarm support is forthcoming from those who could prosper under the new'.

Perhaps the picture is not always as cynical and grim as Machiavelli would suggest. However, there can be little doubt that there are many health care settings where the mere suggestion of primary nursing would be greeted with disbelief, scorn or hostility. Faced in some places with a combination of inadequate nurses, unwilling staff and unsupportive managers or educators, then the prospect of change for primary nursing is indeed daunting. Sometimes presenting a good case can overcome the difficulties (e.g. tapping staff or management support by providing evidence of improved quality of care or better use of resources). At other times, nurses might move elsewhere if that is possible, to settings where their ideas will be received more positively. It is important, however, not to take on all the guilt if nursing does not always go as it might. Nurses often work in poor environments with inadequate resources, behaving in almost a 'heroic' fashion (Lanara, 1981) to maintain standards of care. When this happens, the guilty finger should be pointed quite clearly at the cause of the problem. If nurses fail, maybe it is not always because of weakness in themselves [as they are often made to feel (Salvage, 1985)]; rather, it is in the organisation and how it is governed and resourced that the problem lies. Nurses can help to change things by becoming more aware of the situation, by learning the skills of change agency (skills that can start to be learned on a good interpersonal skills programme) and, not least, by valuing what they do. At the end of a long and hard day (or night), it can seem hopeless to contemplate anything so seemingly remote as primary nursing. But there is a time and place for that. In the meantime, it is important to remember the good things that have been done, to contemplate the benefits, no matter how small, to patients and colleagues that each nurse offers each day – and to cherish them.

CHAPTER 3

The Roles of Nurse and Patient in Primary Nursing

Just as the person who comes to see me needs me for help, I need him to express my ability to give help.

James Hillman
Insearch

Chapter 1 examined some of the central principles of primary nursing. These ideas now need to be developed a little further by looking not only at how the individual roles operate, but at some of the foundations required for the ethos of primary nursing to develop.

VALUING NURSING

Each member of the primary nursing team must value nursing and consider it important, worthwhile and therapeutic. At first sight, this may appear like an overly obvious statement to make, but in many respects nursing could be said to have got its values upside down. Trapped in a culture that espouses the rational, the scientific and the technological – dominated by the hospital-based medical model of care, wrapped up in the higher status associated with cure rather than care – so much of the heart of nursing has become devalued. Many thousands of nurses have come to see themselves in 'the narcissistic mirror offered by medicine' (Oakley, 1984).

Oakley argues that, in order to seek more autonomy, respect and recognition for what they do, nurses have become transfixed by the image in the mirror, not of themselves, but of medicine. In a still largely sexist society, male values predominate, and this is no less true than in male-dominated medicine. The masculine, scientific and rational mode is seen to have more value and status than the (feminine) caring and nurturing mode. Hence the (predominantly female) discipline of nursing has, to a large degree, pursued a false road. By allying itself to high-tech, acute, scientific medicine, it has hoped to gain from some of it status and power. Thus, areas associated with little medical intervention have traditionally had the lower status in nursing (and medicine), e.g. care of the elderly, the mentally handicapped and the mentally ill. The acute sector, associated with high medical intervention, focused on cure, has conversely been awarded higher status. Student nurses tended to gravitate to the latter field after qualification. Nursing has often been described in texts and discussed in classrooms as supportive to medical intervention. 'Basic' nursing is derided as simplistic or common sense – something that can be consigned to junior staff or untrained aides.

I remember being in a room a few years ago discussing allocation of staff in the hospital. A very senior nurse in the acute area commented that all you need in 'geriatrics' is a weak brain and a strong back. I was furious. This was the 1980s. Still this attitude persisted amongst my senior nursing colleagues – 'geriatrics' was good enough for those who weren't too bright, who'd failed their finals, or, worse still, as punishment for those who'd transgressed in the acute sector.

Clinical nurse specialist

Those who aspire to primary nursing recognise at the outset that:

There is no such thing as basic nursing

Those caring, nurturing, 'being with' skills are the very heart of nursing. Whether it be attending to a patient's hygiene, teaching her to walk again, or comforting her when distressed, those activities are not 'basic' or 'menial' (though they are often derided as such); they are skills as valuable, complex and intricate as 'putting up the IVs' or 'giving the medicines as prescribed'.

Lanara (1981) suggests that the nature of so many of what have been put aside as 'basic' tasks are in fact nothing less than heroic acts. She writes:

'In nursing, there are no small and useless tasks. Every little thing counts and every moment weighs, since each is offered for the welfare of human beings. The nurse's work is a composite of significant moments. The high degree of responsibility, the intensity of attention, the alertness of the continuous watching of the critically ill patient, the unpredictability of emergencies, the feverish and laborious task: these are neither exceptions nor recurring cycles. They formulate the everyday rule of the nurse's load. But above and beyond the intensive stress which characterises every single nursing moment, what is known and incomprehensible to many is the heroism of the nurse's heart which, day by day, night by night, creates the unique meanings of nursing. Nursing constitutes an everyday synthesis of all the elements in spiritual grandeur, a grandeur which is inseparable from life's tragedy. Pain and suffering, the tragic element of human life in its greatest intensity and sharpness, constitute the matrix of nursing. And this cannot be transcended without heroism' (Lanara, 1981).

This is not to say that 'high-tech' intervention associated with curative medicine is not part of nursing, rather that it is peripheral to it. The nurse who does not value the heart of nursing, the expressive 'high-touch' role (in both the physical and psychological senses), has rejected nursing in favour of becoming some pseudo-technical assistant. Such a rejection demeans nursing, and turns the nurse into something else – a doctor's handmaiden? a technical servant? a technician? Perhaps all these things and more – anything, but not a nurse. Caring in nursing is healing, in its own right – both separate from, and complementary to, medicine. The nurse who has expanded her role by enhancing, valuing and becoming expert in the 'being with' skills has recognised its therapeutic nature. She might still take on some technical medical task (i.e. use instrumental skills), but only because it is an adjunct to nursing (for example, the community nurse who carries out intravenous injections as *part* of the total care she gives during her visits, to promote a more holistic style of care). However, this person is a very different nurse and holds a very different set of values from the one who takes on such tasks in order to gain some spurious status by seeming to do 'clever' technical-medical functions. One of the challenges for primary nursing is to combine the instrumental and expressive skills, yet retain the essential nature of nursing, which is of value to both nurses and patients.

> We were at a conference discussing the content of the care plans. I remember one nurse in the group being really dismissive of me. She didn't see the point in what I regarded as important care; I mentioned things like 'staying with the patient when he is distressed', 'teaching him how to manage the toilet' and 'getting another nurse to help me lift him'. 'These things are all just common sense', she retorted, and then said: 'Anyway, don't you get bored doing this sort of thing? I do ECGs, take blood, set up drips and things like that. I get far more job satisfaction from this, have a good relationship with my medical colleagues, and should be getting more pay.'
>
> *Clinical nurse specialist*

Within the primary nursing system, nurses have a highly developed set of values of what constitutes nursing. They identify where these roles interlock with other disciplines, but in so doing have a clear image in their heads of what nursing is. Primary nurses work *with* doctors and other disciplines, not *for* them. They work *with* patients and the families and not *at* or *to* them. Nurses immersed in primary nursing have become 'conscious' about nursing. Woods (1987), in explaining the black consciousness movement in South Africa, writes:

'The idea behind Black Consciousness was to break away almost entirely from past black attitudes . . . and to set a new style of self-reliance and dignity for blacks as a psychological attitude leading to new initiatives' (Woods, 1987).

There is a message here for nurses who embark along the road to primary nursing. If the word 'nursing' is transposed at appropriate points in the above quotation, then:

'The idea behind nursing consciousness was to break away almost entirely from past nursing attitudes . . . and to set a new style of self-reliance and dignity for nurses as a psychological attitude leading to new initiatives'.

The 'new initiative' of primary nursing requires more than a commitment to reorganise care; it requires nurses to develop and learn by their beliefs in the value of nursing.

'BEING WITH' THE PATIENT

Nurses involved in primary nursing work on the basis of a new relationship with patients. Wright (1986) and Pearson and Vaughan (1986) speak of 'partnership', and Campbell (1984) of 'companionship'. Both concepts appear to have very similar traits, and Campbell's definition appears to embody the main principles:

'A closeness which is not sexually stereotyped; it implies movement and change; it expresses mutuality; and it requires commitment, but within defined limits . . . companionship describes a closeness which is neither sexual union nor deep personal friendship. It is a bodily presence which accompanies the other for a while. The image of the journey springs to mind when we think of the companions.

Companionship often arises from a chance meeting and it is terminated when the joint purpose which keeps companions together no longer obtains. The good companion is someone who shares freely, but does not impose, allowing others to make their *own* journey' (Campbell, 1984).

Thus primary nurses work with patients, teaching, guiding and advising. They encourage patients to be involved in their own care, to make choices and give information so that the patient can make informed rational decisions. They share their knowledge and skills with the patient. They involve his family, partner and other carers. Where other disciplines are involved, they work with them as part of a team to promote the patient's welfare. When the patient is unable or unwilling to make his wishes known, the primary nurse uses what knowledge is available of him, coupled with empathy skills, to act as his advocate – upholding his wishes when he is unable to do so for himself, advising in his best interests and being prepared to stand accountable for those decisions.

With the above points in mind, perhaps Lathlean (1988) is correct when she asserts that 'Primary nursing can be more stressful than other ways of nursing, and therefore nurses need support to enable them to do the job effectively'. If primary nursing exhorts nurses to become involved with patients, then several profound issues arise.

CAN AND DO ALL NURSES WISH TO BE PRIMARY NURSES?

The answer, quite simply, is no. Firstly, many nurses have not accepted those values of nursing that underlie primary nursing. This issue was covered in some depth earlier in this chapter, and, leaving them aside, there is the question of how far nurses are able to be primary nurses. More attention will be given to the educational preparation of the primary nurse in Chapter 5. Certainly, the present preparation of the nurse leaves much to be desired:

> 'It has been suggested that the roles of registered nurses and sisters are changed by primary nursing. Since we know that nurses are ill-prepared for their existing roles, they are even less likely to be prepared for new ones where, in the case of RGNs, greater autonomy and decision making are required. It could be argued that, when Project 2000 is implemented, this situation will be changed considerably, but it will be a long time before the full effects are felt. Post-basic and continuing educational opportunities vary tremendously across the country, and professional development schemes for registered nurses are only beginning to be offered by health authorities' (Lathlean, 1988).

Benner (1984) further argues that what constitutes the

real nature of nursing is often not taught or valued, and that producing the 'professional' nurse can take many years, certainly more than a basic 3-year programme. A precursor to primary nursing must therefore be the preparation of the nurses. As was suggested in Chapter 2, this might take at least 6 months of further education of the staff, before primary nursing is implemented (more details on suggested content of such preparation are included in Chapter 5). Furthermore it is not just a question of preparation before-hand, but it should be part of a *nursing lifetime* of continuing education and development.

A PRIMARY NURSING CULTURE

Nurses, Menzies (1961) argued, are ill-equipped to cope with the anxiety of the fraught world of nursing and need task allocation to shield them from involvement with the patient. If it is now suggested that nurses become involved, along the lines described by Campbell (1984) as 'companions' or 'partners', how can this challenge be met? If the crutches of task allocation are pulled away, what is needed to replace them so that the nurse does not collapse under the weight of anxiety and stress in her role?

Part of the answer is to equip the nurse with the 'survival skills' (see Chapter 5) that are needed, including assertive-ness and self-awareness. Another part is to develop the climate in which primary nursing and the nurses involved in it can be fostered and nourished. A nursing culture can be produced where the hallmarks are as follows:

- A non-hierarchical, team approach to care.
- Managers and educators are supportive, 'walk the patch', listen to staff views, give praise to reinforce the staff, provide opportunities for further development and support innovation.
- A spirit exists in the team that embodies a 'we are all in this together' approach. Nurses in the team feel free to ask questions and seek advice and support from col-leagues, and are not belittled when they do.
- Change, innovation, research and learning are consi-

dered to be just as important as getting through the work.

● There is an openness, a willingness to share experiences and a flexibility in relationships with colleagues, patients, relatives and others.

● The philosophy of the unit is shared by all; goals and objectives and decisions are jointly agreed.

● The staff place a high value on nursing, and upon holistic and individualised approaches to care.

● Routines and rituals are minimised; the climate supports flexibility in nurse–patient activities.

It could be argued that factors such as these should be the norm in any nursing setting, and indeed this is so! Unfortunately, many nurses do not experience such benefits (Price Waterhouse, 1988). A primary nursing culture is essential to the creation and maintenance of primary nursing and to the welfare of both patients and staff involved in it.

> I remember as a student being 'ticked off' for sitting talking with a patient. 'Haven't you anything to do?', I was asked. It's not like that here. I have my patients. If talking with them is part of their needs, then I get on with it. The team here know what nursing is. They've got their priorities right.
>
> *Primary nurse*

AUTONOMY AND ACCOUNTABILITY

Making decisions about care, being free to carry them out, and accepting responsibility for the effects underpin the role of the primary nurse. However, as Bergman (1981) points out, professional freedom to this degree means that nurses must have the ability to make such decisions and to take on such responsibility as well as having the authority to pursue them. The bureaucratic nature of much of health care and the status of nursing within it leaves nurses in a very hazy position.

Dimond (1988), as a barrister with a particular interest and expertise in nursing issues, has argued that, in law, nursing care essentially remains within the domain of the doctor. Recent trends, however, have been pushing the nurse further and further along the road to professional autonomy and accountability. The Code of Professional Conduct and Project 2000 (UKCC, 1983 and 1986 respectively) envisage a nurse who is directly accountable to the patient.

There can be little doubt that nurses who assert professional autonomy and choose to accept their accountability are skating on the thin ice at the outer edges of the profession. Some nurses (for example, those who raised objections to electroconvulsive therapy) have found this to their cost.

In practice, the legal position is very unclear and often ill-considered by nurses. At the same time, fears over litigation are often thrown up as an excuse for not changing, or for not trying anything new. Primary nursing is about putting into action what is in effect a worldwide nursing phenomenon – the desire for professional self-determination. It is certain that the legal framework in which this is carried out needs to be clarified to remove the uncertainty from nurses and the attendant sense of risk.

While many fears over 'What happens if . . .?' may surface in nurses from time to time, such risks need to be set in perspective. The reality is that most nurses work well in team relationships with colleagues, and problems that get to the point of litigation are relatively minimal. This is not to underestimate the importance of the issue, rather to set it more realistically in context.

We decided to press on with our plans to let the patients have access to their nursing plans. We agreed as a team and kept other colleagues, including the doctors, informed. It's worked well, but part of the reason seems to be us, the way we work together here. I know someone who tried the same idea in another place, and it was squashed before it even got off the ground. He was given all kinds of legal reasons why it wouldn't work, and one doctor refused permission anyway. So, it never happened – 'too dangerous', he was told. I ask you, if nurses worked on that basis all the time, you'd never get past your front door! I often think that the relationship you build up with colleagues, so that you are trusted and respected, is as important as any legal framework. I know what I am and how to do it, and am quite prepared to stand up and be counted

continued next page

continued

if I drop a clanger! I do not need someone else to *permit* me to decide what nursing is, though I understand in law that's strictly speaking the doctor's prerogative. Well, laws change, customs and practice change. I'd rather we led the way on this than sat forever under the doctor's coat-tails or hid behind the hospital procedure book! We work well here, we've a collegiate relationship that works, and it works because we each know where the other stands, and what each other's jobs are.

Senior primary nurse/ward sister

Nurses who set out on primary nursing are, to some degree, pursuing a professional adventure. If they take on the perceptions of autonomy to practise and accountability to the patient, they must also take on board the implications that go with them. Not only are there greater freedoms in decision-making about nursing practice, there are also greater responsibilities (of keeping up to date, of maintaining high standards, of practising on the basis of sound knowledge, of being prepared to be accountable, and so on) which go with them.

THE ROLES

This chapter concludes with a brief outline of the principal roles in primary nursing and how they work with patients (and others) in the revised way discussed above. Throughout the literature on primary nursing, there are three key roles envisaged: primary nurse, associate nurse and care assistant. How far each of these roles fits with the principal existing clinical jobs in the UK, e.g. sister/charge nurse/ staff nurse/enrolled nurse/nursing auxiliary/assistant, will be discussed in more detail in Chapter 4.

The Primary Nurse

The primary nurse is seen as a registered (first level) nurse, having undertaken at least a 3-year programme of education. This is the key role responsible for assessing, planning, implementing and evaluating the care of the patient from admission through to discharge or transfer. This nurse is accountable for the care that is prescribed and given, and may have added responsibilities in teaching, researching and managing others in the nursing team involved in the patient's care. The primary nurse co-ordinates the patient's nursing care, as well as liaising with other members of the multidisciplinary team to ensure that it is comprehensive. This includes working with relatives, visitors and others. The primary nurse might be seen as sitting at the centre of the web of care with the patient, working as a partner and companion in care, and pulling together all the many strands involved in his health and well-being. The primary nurse is knowledgeable and autonomous, basing practice on sound rationale, yet seeking help, advice and further self-development to ensure that the practice is up to date. The primary nurse works with colleagues, using a nursing model to generate nursing practice, and participates in the evaluation of care in the wider sphere, for example in quality assurance programmes to ensure that the delivery of care is of the highest quality.

The primary nurse prepares the patient for discharge and joins in the multidisciplinary team decision on this issue. In some units, such as the Burford and Oxford Nursing Units (Pearson, 1988b), the primary nurse may also have designated 'nursing beds' where medical intervention is relatively small. The primary nurse may control the admission and discharge of patients in these beds. Having nursing beds, however, is not essential to primary nursing.

The Associate Nurse

This nurse need not necessarily be a registered nurse (although the primary nurse can 'act across' for a colleague's patients and care for them as an associate nurse in her absence). The associate nurse cares for the patient in the absence of the primary nurse, and may adjust the care as necessary. Major changes are carried out in consultation with the primary nurse. In some settings, this may mean that the primary nurse may work 'on call' or suggest that she can be contacted even when off duty if a particular issue of importance crops up. In practice, these should only be on rare occasions. Where the associate nurse is not a registered nurse, then other registered (primary) nurses must be on site to monitor the patients' care and offer help and guidance if needed. Continuity of care is essential and must be backed up by written care plans and effective verbal reporting methods. The associate nurse works very closely with the primary nurse to co-ordinate the patient's care and contribute to a rich information exchange, so that all facets of the patient's care can be constantly monitored and evaluated.

In the absence of the primary nurse, the associate nurse remains accountable in his or her own right and can adjust the plan of care accordingly. Primary nursing does not mean that the associate nurse must not do anything unless the primary nurse has made the decision.

The Care Assistant

These assistants help the primary nurses and associate nurses by carrying out the non-nursing duties essential to the order of a unit. They may assist the primary and associate nurses in the giving of care (e.g. helping them to bath a patient or helping with lifting or exercises). They may help, for example, with the preparation and serving of meals, with bed-making and with the general orderliness and upkeep of the ward. Although not a trained nurse, the care assistant is included with others as part of the nursing team and is expected to contribute to decisions about the unit as well as to offer observations on patients and their progress in the overall evaluation of the patient's care.

> The primary nurse is responsible for making a plan of care for each patient in our group, and my job is to work with these patients and nurse for the whole of my shift, helping to give the care planned for them.
>
> I am always fully informed of their condition. I get a full verbal report and can have an input to their care planning, e.g. reporting on bowel movements or incontinence episodes, etc. I can contribute to the hand-over report for these

continued next page

continued

patients and tell the staff about any changes I've observed. This information is always listened to, and is of value to trained staff in planning the nursing care. We work closely as a team and have regular meetings for discussions, and all staff participate. I sit in on case conferences held for the patient and am made to feel my judgment is trusted and valued.

I assist my nurse with patient care – washing, dressing, toiletting, etc., as well as seeing to the general orderliness of the ward. By working as a member of a small team looking after a small group of patients, I am left time to do other activities with them – letter writing, crossword puzzles or hairstyling – or simply just talking with and listening to them.

Primary nursing has meant that I now have the time and the opportunity to build up a good and sometimes quite close relationship with the patients. I find it more rewarding to be with both patients and staff in this way.

The care assistant has a significant role to play in supporting primary nursing. He or she needs to feel fully involved as part of the team, and should also be given opportunities for education and personal development to help them fulfil it to the maximum.

Care assistant

The above provides a general outline of the main roles, and clearly there is a need for co-ordination of these activities. The role of the ward sister/charge nurse remains 'key' (Pembrey, 1980) in this respect. More details of these organisational matters are discussed in Chapter 4.

Nursing is a healing presence with patients, and this chapter has sought to develop further areas on how primary nursing can enhance that presence as well as look at some of the concerns for the nurses and patients involved. This type of involvement requires considerable skill and commitment, and yet more, for it is not too grand a word to use to suggest that it takes 'love', a 'moderated love' (Campbell, 1984) that helps both nurse and patient to find their way through the complexity of their relationship and dependence on each other. This love requires respect for the individual on the part of the nurse, a genuine desire to help another human being in what might, at the very least, be difficult and distressing times. Nurses are frequently called upon to transmit this love, often against great odds of poor staffing levels and resources. When they fail to do so, they can feel

bad about themselves, even though their lack of prepared-
ness, of support, of resources, is the real root of the problem.
Nurses involved in primary nursing are tapping that love in
the often heroic effort to do what is best for the patient. It is a
love which rests on the recognition of the value of nursing
and of the nurse, for the nurse who does not love him or
herself will not be able to offer it in turn to the patient. Care
without the component of this moderated form of love is like
wine without the alcohol – there is something missing; it
may look the same, but it does not *feel* the same.

Primary nursing thus demands much of its nurses, but it
has the potential to give so much to them and their patients
in return. Many contentious issues and problems have so far
been raised, and in the next chapter we will look at how some
of these can be resolved.

CHAPTER 4

Organisational Matters
– Twenty Questions!

People will tell you where they've gone,
They'll tell you where to go
But till you get there yourself, you never really know

Joni Mitchell (1976)
Amelia
From the album 'Hejira' on Asylum Records

Every setting, every nurse, is unique. Thus, all the contributors to this text are wary of being prescriptive. From the experience of dealing with the thousands of visitors who have been to Tameside's Nursing Development Unit, the kind of questions and concerns raised by nurses tend to be very similar. Often what nurses seek is a magic box, filled with all the right answers: 'Give me your box that I may go away and do likewise!'

The principles of primary nursing are universal but the application is open to many options. Flexibility is the key. Anything that nurses do to make care more personal, often in very difficult circumstances, needs to be valued and cherished, whether it is full-blown primary nursing or not. Indeed there are many simple acts – a shift in the ward routine here, an adjustment to the usual ritual there – that nurses can accomplish without a great deal of effort or resources to improve the lot of both patients and nurses. Sometimes it is difficult to judge which comes first – a climate of hope and innovation from which primary nursing is but a natural step, or primary nursing (or just thinking about it) which sets the ball of innovative practice rolling.

Whichever is the case (and it is probably a combination of both), experience has confirmed what has been suggested in the previous chapters – there comes a time. It is difficult to describe or measure. It is intangible, qualitative and intuitive, but a time comes when a place is ripe for primary nursing – that peculiar combination of circumstances of people and the place that transforms the situation beyond 'on your marks' to 'get set, then go'.

The rest of this chapter is therefore devoted not only to answering some of the very common questions that arise when nurses embark on primary nursing, but also to dealing with the problems and questions that arise once the process is under way. The questions here deal principally with the 'doing' of primary nursing and are set in no particular order of priority.

1. What Happens to the Role of the Ward Sister/Charge Nurse?

In short it undergoes a radical transformation from the traditional role, i.e. that of total controller of the nursing team and their actions. Primary nursing is about the unleashing of the individual autonomy and accountability of each primary nurse. It is incompatible with rigid, autocratic, hierarchical forms of nursing, whether in hospital or the community.

> The sister or charge nurse is still the key figure, but in different ways. Primary nursing will not work unless he or she lets it. The role changes dramatically, new roles are taken on and some old ones discarded.
>
> *Senior primary nurse/charge nurse*

If each primary nurse is to practise with autonomy, the role of the ward sister remains 'key' (Pembrey, 1980) to the success. However, primary nursing is not a charter for anarchy. Nurses operate on very different levels of experience and knowledge of nursing (Benner, 1984), and it is the ward sister or charge nurse who has developed to the level of expert who acts as the support to colleagues. Some of these nurses will have achieved this level of expertise and can then be given full reign for their autonomy, the sister/charge nurse acting as the support person to enable them to get on with the job. For others, a higher degree of monitoring and supervision may be needed to ensure that all clinical decisions are accurate and safe. This can produce a dilemma for the clinical team and there is a danger here of giving conflicting signals (on the one hand letting go, on the other checking up on what nurses do). Ultimately, how well this works depends upon the strength of the team, the nature of the collegiate relationship and the degree of trust embodied between colleagues. It is these that ensure that the managerial powers of the sister/charge nurse are used and interpreted in the team not as, 'I'm in charge and I'm watching what you're doing because I'm unsure of you or you're not experienced enough', but as, 'Because of my experience and the authority I've been given, I'm here to help you, support you and guide you in your practice so that both you and the patient don't come to harm'.

The difference in style is distinct, but subtle, and there is no underestimating the interpersonal skills this key person must have to do it effectively. Primary nursing, while fostering autonomy, is not an unbridled licence for all nurses to act without question or supervision. Not all nurses have achieved the level of expert; not all have total awareness of the limitations to their knowledge and skill. The working relationship between the team leader – the sister/charge nurse – will vary with each member of that team according to their unique qualities. Encouraging primary nurses towards autonomy does not mean that the team leader abrogates his or her role as professional adviser, monitor and co-ordinator of care (Figure 4.1).

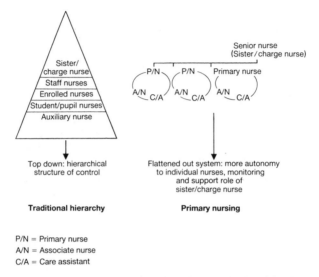

Fig. 4.1   The changed nature of the team relationship in primary nursing. (After Sparrow, 1986)

I have to be sure of myself as a clinical practitioner and manager to take on the role. My ward does not lend itself to my being a primary nurse, I leave that to the others. I have chosen to work as an associate nurse. I see myself as the lynch-pin on the ward, yet at the same time I have to be able to devolve responsibility and decision making. I have to let them get on with it yet be there to support them and make sure that all decisions and actions are the right ones. It doesn't mean I'm breathing down their necks all the time – we wouldn't have primary nursing if that were the case. It's more subtle than that, difficult to explain, but you *know* when it's working. I think in part, you get there when the staff see you as a sort of nursing consultant. You know you're on the right track when the self-awareness (in part developed by you) is such that they approach *you* for help because they know they are at the limits of their knowledge or skill.

Senior primary nurse/charge nurse

The effects of this shift of role for the 'captain of the team' vary according to the current style the sister/charge nurse already used. In some it is a natural development; for others it can be a radical shift, an almost terrifying experience.

> I found that I needed peer support too. I have to support everybody else, but what about me! The support of management and colleagues is crucial. You go through all kinds of feelings, because you're brought up to be in control, to be 'in charge'. You feel uncomfortable at first, a bit insecure, and have to be wary of rushing to the defences and getting authoritarian again. It just takes time, you work through it.
>
> *Senior primary nurse/ward sister*

The role of the ward sister/charge nurse, therefore, undergoes considerable changes with primary nursing. From being the 'head of the ward, fount of all knowledge, decisions not be questioned' figure, he or she becomes the 'navigator' of the ward or unit, giving it direction and a sense of cohesion. The roles as counsellor, facilitator, supporter, teacher and researcher are enhanced (roles which the sister/charge nurse is expected to fulfil anyway) and come more to the fore. Indeed, freed of 'total control', the sister/charge nurse has the time to give to these functions, and to be a more effective manager and user of the resources of the unit.

> I had to become a counsellor, teacher, guide all in one. I saw it as my job to create the climate where we could all grow as a team, express views and seek advice freely without anxiety or fear of recrimination. We have regular meetings – planned and ad-hoc, social gatherings, and working groups looking into certain topics. I delegated all kinds of things to the others, one primary nurse looking after the off-duty, another monitoring the holidays, someone else to keep an eye on the stocks and stores. We set up a quality circle. Individual nurses were designated as 'information seekers' when a topic or problem came up, to report back to the whole team on their findings; others meanwhile were encouraged to become the ward 'mini' specialist, for example one for continence advice, another for pressure area care. All these ideas were really to get over to the team that responsibilities were devolved.
>
> *Senior primary nurse/charge nurse*

The sister/charge nurse has a key role to play too, in developing both self and colleagues, keeping up to date by reading journals, attending courses and conferences, and so on, as an inherent part of primary nursing (as it should be in all aspects of nursing!). The team leader has the task of fostering the development not only of him/herself, but also of colleagues in the team. Without a sense of continuous learning and development, primary nursing can shrivel up.

2. Can the Sister/Charge Nurse be a Primary Nurse?

Yes, in both hospital and community settings. In the community, where the nurse works on a one-to-one basis with patients and families, this is relatively straightforward. (Indeed, some community nurses would agree that they have always been primary nurses.) In hospitals or nursing homes dealing with larger groups of staff, then many alternatives are available depending on the individual characteristics (patient dependency, skill mix, staffing levels, etc.) of each setting, for example:

- Sister/charge nurse takes full caseload of patients (equal to other primary nursing colleagues).
- Takes reduced caseload as primary nurse while focusing on other duties.
- Does not act as primary nurse but as an associate nurse to a specific primary nurse.
- Acts neither as associate nor primary nurse, but remains free to deal with other activities, or 'floats', and takes over as associate or primary nurse (e.g. during sickness or absence of associate nurse or primary nurse).

Lathlean (1988) is of the view that:

'The sister, unless acting as a primary nurse, does not prescribe or actually give care. She acts as the co-ordinator of nursing staff, a resource and information provider and, importantly support giver – a role which differs greatly from that of the traditional sister.

In practice, the person occupying this role may be given an alternative title to highlight the differences. Some health authorities are developing senior roles, known as senior sisters, where the occupant is responsible for the management of a ward's nursing budget, decisions about skill mix of nursing staff and the provision of expert advice, without day-to-day account-ability for the care of individual patients'.

Whichever of the above, or combinations of them, is chosen must depend on a flexible approach depending on the qualities of the particular unit. Depending on the level of commitment as primary nurse, the sister/charge nurse can act as overall co-ordinator of the ward. In other instances, the primary nurses may share this load and rotate ward co-ordinating functions amongst themselves. Whichever is the case, it is important that the sister or charge nurse remains a clinician in order to be an effective role model, whether it be as primary nurse or associate nurse.

3. Who is the Primary Nurse?

There is general agreement that the primary nurse must be a first level registered nurse, as has been suggested earlier. This is based on a combination of factors (preparation during training, legal responsibilities, codes of conduct, etc.). However, as Benner (1984) has noted, there can be a great variety in the expertise of individual nurses, and Manthey (1970) notes how 'Experience as well as education must be taken into account when assessing an individual nurse's level of expertise in caring for various levels of patients.' It may well be that in terms of knowledge, skill and experience, an individual enrolled nurse might be better equipped to deliver a patient's care than a newly qualified RGN. The position of the enrolled nurse will be dealt with below. The primary nurse, meanwhile, requires a rolling programme of support and professional development to achieve the level of expert in care. It must run in parallel with the nurse's gradual development in practice, so that, over time, the primary nurse gradually achieves competence as expert autonomous practitioner.

4. What about the Enrolled Nurse?

Having two levels of qualified nurse in British nursing has produced many problems, and primary nursing forces a confrontation with some of these issues. In principle, the primary nurse is a first level registered nurse. Yet many settings have a higher dependency on enrolled nurses (and would have difficulty in recruiting otherwise). Where the enrolled nurse is used as primary nurse, then a number of factors need to be considered:

- What is happening is not primary nursing; it is something else – a more advanced form of patient allocation perhaps, but not, strictly speaking, primary nursing.
- The enrolled nurse him/herself, without pressure, agrees with being a primary nurse, and this is done on the basis of informed consent, i.e. he/she has been fully informed about primary nursing, in particular the knowledge and skills needed and the relationship to accountability, and is therefore still willing to take on the role.
- The enrolled nurse has been adequately prepared for the role.
- The unit's staff and management are in agreement on the issue, and this agreement is fully documented.

> It needs to be mentioned that this issue must be handled delicately if the enrolled nurse is not to feel that she is not trusted. It requires a degree of understanding and mutual support amongst the staff and a recognition that these precautions are taken, not because 'we don't trust the SEN' but because we need to ensure that she is adequately supported and covered in the unlikely event of something going wrong.
>
> *Primary nurse*

It has been argued that when the enrolled nurse takes on the role, the legal framework is somewhat doubtful. It is also worth noting that if the enrolled nurse is skilled enough to act as a primary nurse, then he/she should be fully educated (e.g. offered a conversion course) and paid as such.

There is no doubting the very real dilemma surrounding the role of the enrolled nurse (EN) in primary nursing, particularly in settings where they are a large part of the nursing workforce. Some of these aspects therefore need also to be considered:

● The primary nurse role (the word 'primary' has a ring of higher status or importance about it) should not be sold at the expense of the other roles.

When we explained to the ENs what primary nursing was all about, a lot of rethinking went on. It is absolutely essential to ensure that the associate nurse role (which seemed to us to be a more appropriate role for the EN) is *valued*. I can't stress this enough. It's an important part of the whole approach, so you can't afford to have people feeling they occupy some second rate role. Taking this approach, most of our SENs have been happy in this capacity.

Nurse manager

Valuing the role of the associate nurse is a vital step in removing problems over status or of feeling devalued. This must happen within the whole team in order to develop the right niche for the enrolled nurse who chooses not to be a primary nurse.

● A strategy (and it may well be a long-term one) might need to be developed for revising the skill mix in a unit (see Chapter 6), gradually helping more enrolled nurses to undertake conversion courses (if they wish to do it) and steadily increasing the proportion of first level registered nurses to other grades of staff.

5. What about Staffing Levels and Skill Mixes?

According to Watson (1978) these must be *adequate* and *consistent*. She recommends the following:

Patients per primary nurse	Type of care
2	Critical care unit
5	Acute
7	Long term

Thus on a ward of 25 acutely ill patients, there would need to be at least 5 RGNs (full time) acting as primary nurses, with sufficient numbers of associate nurses (Watson argues for 2·5 per primary nurse) and care assistants to continue the care in the absence of the primary nurse. In addition to the number of staff, getting the skill mix right can be a difficult issue and may be the subject of longer term planning before primary nursing begins (see Chapter 2). The problems here can be aggravated by local recruitment difficulties, the popularity/unpopularity of the specialty, and so on. However, the experience of some units (Pearson, 1988a; Purdy et al, 1988) suggests that moves towards primary nursing can enhance staff recruitment so that the desired skill mix can be achieved. This appears to support the findings of other research (McClure et al, 1983; Price Waterhouse, 1988) that nurses are attracted to areas in which they feel they can practise nursing with greater autonomy and freedom.

> We wanted to do primary nursing years ago, but with 80% of the workforce untrained it seemed a pipe-dream. Over the years, we've adjusted the mix as people have left – now we have 65% trained staff, and the pipe-dream can be a reality.
>
> *Consultant nurse and nurse manager*

There is still much debate relating to appropriate skill mix of nurses in relation to patient dependency, partly because so much of nursing is difficult to measure, as is the quality of care delivered. Watson's paper, cited above, must be taken as very generalised figures that can be used as a basis for agreeing staffing levels and mixes. In some units (e.g. intensive care or the critically ill patient on the general ward), a one-to-one relationship may be necessary. Other writers have indicated greater variations in these figures [up to 11 or 12 patients per primary nurse in continuing care settings (Hegyvary, 1982; Tutton, 1986)].

> On our unit, we found that five or six patients per primary nurse is a comfortable ratio, and with very little variation between the acute and continuing care wards. That's not to say that the primary nurse looks after her
>
> *continued next page*

continued

patients and no others. Sometimes the primary nurse can act as an associate nurse for another primary nurse. The ward sister only takes a caseload of one or two patients, and the rest of the back-up team make up the total number of staff on the ward.

Primary nurse

The total number of staff on the ward must reflect the individual characteristics of the setting, and as yet no completely reliable tools for making calculations have emerged.

The skill mix change was most important to us; what we found was that quality, not quantity, matters. There are fewer 'bodies' on the ward, in terms of the total number of staff, but practice is much more autonomous, i.e. I wouldn't have to waste my time supervising numbers of untrained staff.

Primary nurse

As MacGuire (1988) succinctly points out: 'The exact values of staff at different levels may be less important largely because of the great variability on a day to day basis at ward level. What does matter is that we look at what is happening at the ward level and make the most of the skills and abilities which are there'.

6. How are Patients Allocated to Nurses?

In some instances, allocation of patients is made by the most senior nurse (head nurse or ward sister/charge nurse), otherwise by mutual agreement of the primary nurses. The choice should be made by the staff on site. Varying lengths of stay of patients, staffing levels and skill mixes may mean that the number of patients per primary nurse may vary even within one unit. Assessment on the basis of the scope of patients' needs, not just physical status, is the determining factor. In addition, the patient may wish to have a say in who his or her primary nurse might be.

In some areas it might be possible to work out a 'take' rota, e.g. patients are allocated to nurses as they are admitted to a unit, with nurses taking it in turns both on a daily or shift-by-shift basis.

> We find, quite simply, that letting the staff determine the allocation of patients is a team decision. If a problem arises, then the charge nurse can always step in to make the decision if agreement cannot be reached, but in practice this never happened.
>
> *Senior primary nurse/charge nurse*

In the agreement, the principle should be that each patient should be able to identify his or her nurse for however long or short a time the patient's problem requires nursing care. Whether the patient arrives as a day case on the ward or is resident in a coronary care setting, or is requiring a limited number of visits in the community, then the goal is to achieve the 'my nurse' concept.

7. How Does the Nurse Make Herself Known to the Patient and Explain Primary Nursing?

Apart from the obvious point of introducing oneself and explaining to the patient what primary nursing is all about, there are additional factors that can enhance patients' awareness of what is going on. After all, the patient may be disorientated or, with so many other things going on in his/her life at the time of illness in an unfamiliar setting, simply forgetful. In addition, other people need to know too: relatives, visitors, doctors, physiotherapists and the other disciplines who visit the ward. Wills and Wright (1988) identified the following possible features:

- The use of 'business cards' (Figure 4.2), which can be given to patients or relatives.

FRONT:

The Nursing Development Unit

Telephone:
Ask for Ward . . . .

. . . .
Primary Nurse   Associate Nurse

Caring for the Elderly

REVERSE:

You can expect your primary nurse to:
Get to know you and your family.
Plan with your doctor, for your care.
Plan with you the nursing care, to meet your needs.
Explain your needs to the associate nurse, who will care for you when your primary nurse is off duty.
Tell you what to expect before all tests or treatment.
Teach you about health care related to your condition.
Find the answers to your questions about your hospital stay.

We need you to:
Tell your primary nurse what you need.
Keep your nurse informed about how you feel and things that are on your mind.
Let your nurse know how you feel about the care you receive.
Tell your nurse if you have an idea or a preference about your nursing care.

Fig. 4.2   Example of a business card

> We have also produced identification cards for the primary nurses. We use a modification of the system used at Emory University Hospital, Atlanta (the link hospital in our international exchange system). The patient has one of these but they are useful for relatives too, to identify the nurse and provide an easy reference for the ward's telephone number.
>
> To start with, these are not particularly cheap to produce (about £170 per 3000 including artwork, etc.) but thereafter they cost about £30 per 1000. We consider this a worthwhile investment if it initiates understanding between nurse, patient and others and makes contact easier.
>
> *Primary nurse*

- At the entrance to the ward, a notice-board can be set up that gives the names of the patients, their location on the ward, and the names of the primary/associate nurses caring for them. Photographs of the nursing staff, with names, can also be on display.
- Each ward can have an information centre for the use of both patients and relatives. Articles and information on primary nursing can be made available for staff, patients and relatives to read. Information leaflets (Figure 4.3) for visitors to collect as they wish, can also be made available.

- Another possibility is to have photographs of nurse and patient at the bedside:

> At the bedside on the continuing care wards, it is possible to have a photograph of both nurse and patient together, which can be attached to the head of the bed. This is not so easy on rapid turnover wards, but here we have found that simply a photograph of the nurse is sufficient. At the side of the picture is a name label giving the details of patient, primary nurse and associate nurse.
>
> *Primary nurse*

- Information books can also be given to patients.

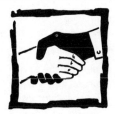

The Nursing Development Unit

Dear Visitor

Primary Nursing – what does it mean?

The Nursing Staff on the Ward would like to tell you about a new approach to nursing our patients – it's called 'Primary Nursing'.

Each patient has his or her own special nurse, called a 'Primary Nurse', who is the main person looking after the patient. An 'Associate Nurse' helps the Primary Nurse to give the care required.

When you visit our ward, look out for a photo of the 'Primary Nurse' with her 'Special Patient' and the information card telling you the name of the 'Special Nurse'. These are placed over the bed and on the notice board as you enter the ward.

For information about the patient you are visiting, or about Primary Nursing, please ask the Primary Nurse, who is the main care giver, or the Associate Nurse if she is not on duty. You might like to make a note of the two special nurses, so that you can ask for them if making a telephone enquiry.

We always welcome any comments regarding the nursing care of our patients: please let the Primary Nurse know your views.

Thank you
The Nursing Staff

Caring for the Elderly

Fig. 4.3 Example of an information leaflet

Each patient is given an information booklet. Apart from giving details on a variety of issues pertinent to his hospital stay, there is also a section describing primary nursing. The following is an extract from the booklet:

Nursing Care. As often as possible the same nurses will be caring for you during your stay on the ward, so that you can get to know them and they can get to know you. You may be allocated your own special nurse, known as a 'primary nurse', who will be responsible for your nursing care throughout your stay. Your care will be discussed with you, and you are encouraged to read your nursing notes if you wish to. You will be asked if you would like your nursing notes to be kept at the bedside, or if you would prefer them to be kept at the nurses' station.

Associate nurse

The above suggestions are not substitutes for effective nurse/patient communication, but they do help to support it. Above all, as Manthey (1970) suggests, the primary nurse is a 'visible' nurse who is known to the patient, the family and other disciplines.

8. What about Day-to-Day Organisation?

McFarlane and Castledine (1982) describe the pattern of care they used in one unit, which includes the following:

1. Each patient is allocated to a primary nurse for:
    - assessing, planning, implementing and evaluating care
    - working with patients each time he/she is on duty
    - following patients' progress through hospitalisation
    - making home visits, e.g. before, during and after discharge
    - arranging transfer home
    - functioning as the patients' advocate
    - serving as the main co-ordinator of his total care
    - promoting his care at nursing care evaluation sessions.
2. Each patient is also allocated to a second (associate) nurse/student/nursing auxiliary, who helps to continue

care both when the primary nurse is present and when she is away.

3. All nurses serve as associates to each other in the event of both primary and other associate nurse being absent.
4. Primary nurses attend case conferences, ward rounds, etc., when possible.
5. Primary nurse discusses changes with plan after days off, etc.
6. One nurse acts as overall ward co-ordinator on each shift (not necessarily ward sister).

The above illustrates one general approach to the organisation of primary nursing. Co-ordinating the staff in this way raises new difficulties. 'Off-duties' can be planned to ensure that 'care' is provided by both associate and primary nurse on rotation. These might actually look different from the usual 'off-duty' sheet (e.g. Figure 4.4).

In the example given in Figure 4.4, individual off-duties are organised to ensure sufficient 'cover' of staff and skill mixes during the course of the day. In other words, the off-duty is planned to ensure general trained staff cover of a particular unit, as well as ensuring that each group of patients retains their primary and associate nurses. Reorganising care along the lines of primary nursing can also bring about a change in the overall pattern of the patient's day. Traditionally, staffing levels tend to be planned with higher numbers in the morning and fewer in the evening. This may shift with primary nursing.

We used to have six staff on in the morning and three or four in the evening (large, long-stay care of the elderly ward). Now, with the change of skill mix and the change in the pattern of the day, we need the numbers to be much more even – say 4/4 or 5/4.

Senior primary nurse/ward sister

Changing the shift levels in one ward can, however, cause problems.

WARD DUTY ROTA   **WARD:**   **WEEK COMMENCING:**

Name	Monday	Tuesday	Wednesday	Thursday	Friday	Saturday	Sunday
Primary nurse							
Associate nurse							
Associate nurse							
Care assistant							
Primary nurse							
Associate nurse							
Associate nurse							
Care assistant							
Primary nurse							
Associate nurse							
Associate nurse							
Care assistant							
Primary nurse							
Associate nurse							
Associate nurse							
Care assistant							
Total ward numbers							

Fig. 4.4   'Off-duty' sheet

Our ward ratios were different, but other wards working to the old pattern stayed the same. When someone went off sick (on the other wards), we began to feel like the loan-shop for the rest of the unit, i.e. we were seen to have higher than usual numbers of staff in the evening but, of course, they were there because they were needed. Other staff in other wards, though, can perceive you as being well off and therefore available for borrowing from.

Primary nurse

Another possibility to consider is flexible rostering. This can work on some units where the caseload is more erratic. For example, a surgical ward may organise their staff's hours to deal with planned admissions.

> I've been to one ward where they take lots of day cases. Some of the primary nurses took it in turns to adjust their hours, working from the time the patient came in, staying with them throughout their care during the day, until they went home. With flexible hours, they took the time back later.
>
> *Associate nurse*

In organising the day-to-day work of the ward, a variety of strategies can be tried as different options. In the end, what suits a particular setting best is that with which all staff and patients feel comfortable, and this can only be decided on an individual basis.

9. What about Borrowing of Staff?

Primary nursing does not guarantee that nurses will not go off sick or that staffing crises do not occur (although it is argued that such incidents are reduced).

There can be problems when primary nursing is being implemented in some areas and not others.

> Our off-duties changed, that is the spread of staff over the day became different. We didn't have more staff, just deployed them differently. This meant we used to have three staff on duty in the evening where now we have four. The trouble is, other wards can see us as well staffed if their numbers fall. The pressure is on the borrower. They don't realise that the four staff are there because they are needed.
>
> *Primary nurse*

Primary nursing need not mean that staff become inflexible or unresponsive to the wider sense of the team which exists on the larger unit. Helping each other out is an essential consequence when problems arise. However, it does place an issue firmly before management: look at a whole range of strategies to reduce the problem and not just manage the crisis by shunting staff around.

> I had a terrible incident one evening. It left me quaking in my shoes! The nurse manager wanted to borrow one of my staff. I didn't refuse at first and tried to get him to look at how we could help without major depletion of our staff (i.e. we could have adjusted our working pattern in the short term to help 'cover' for meals, etc.). In the end, I had to point out the care planning and the allocation of patients, and the workload. I told him, 'If you take this primary nurse, then six patients will have no-one to care for them. Would you please sign in the notes that you will accept responsibility if anything goes wrong or if there is a complaint!'. I told him that 'We will cope if we have to, I can't *stop* you enforcing your decision, but if you do, I want it in writing'. I thought, this is it – the sack! He went white and just left the ward. Then I felt really awful, not just for myself, but for the other ward which I knew must be really stuck, but I told myself: 'My priority is my patients, my code of conduct tells me that there's no point in robbing Peter to pay Paul'. How did it end? He called someone in on overtime!
>
> *Senior primary nurse/ward sister*

Borrowing and moving of staff has become an accepted activity in nursing because nurses will 'cope'. It should be seen as a last resort when all other strategies have failed. It is not a problem unique to primary nursing, and it is short changing patients wherever and whenever it occurs. What primary nursing seems to do is to thrust the difficulty into sharp focus. When considered with the skills of the questioning assertive nurse, then the manager's role is also tested. Is support for primary nursing merely lip-service or is there really a creative management approach evident? Issues like staffing problems are one of the ways in which this is tested.

It also has to be said that the borrowing of staff does not mean that primary nursing has collapsed. In the short term, it may be no more than an irritant or frustration that niggles at the clinical nurse who has to work around it. However, if it becomes consistent and long term, it may undermine the whole practice of primary nursing, which depends at least upon a reasonably reliable deployment of staff. Primary nurses and their colleagues cannot continue in their role when they are dogged by constant uncertainties of who their patients will be. The expectations of the patients are also not fulfilled in such circumstances. The occasional 'slip' in staffing levels – a ward or small unit when staff and patients are well known to each other – can easily be managed. If it becomes a permanent problem, it must be questioned whether effort to maintain primary nursing can be continued, because of the risks of exhaustion and frustration to the staff and the conflicting messages being given to patients. In the long term, primary nursing requires reasonable stability in the nursing workforce. When this is not happening, then questions must be asked, beyond primary nursing, about what is going wrong that keeps nurses out of commitment to nursing, and what can be done to put things right.

10. What Reporting Methods are Necessary?

If the basis of primary nursing is that of a working partnership with the patient, then this will require a shift away from traditional reporting methods (i.e. the staff gathered separately from patients at 'hand-over' time). In the Nursing Development Unit at Tameside the following methods have proved effective:

- Each primary or associate nurse gives a verbal and written report on his/her group of patients.
- All staff are involved in a general 'walk round' of the ward at report hand-over times (e.g. between two shifts) to receive the verbal report. This ensures that all staff have a working knowledge of all patients. They can still therefore render effective help to all patients, e.g. in the sudden absence of the primary/associate nurse or simply 'in passing'. Primary nursing does not mean that the allocated nurses attend only to 'my patients' and ignore all others! The staff still have to work as a team.
- Patients' nursing records are kept at the bedside (if they choose) and reports are made with the patient at the

bedside. The patient may write in the notes if he or she wishes. Of course, the patient will not be disturbed for note writing while asleep.

- The patient is involved in discussion on his or her care at report times by the team. These tend to be very general discussions so that confidentiality is not breached within earshot of the patients. Detailed aspects of care can be discussed separately between individual nurses transferring care of the patient, and between nurse and patient.
- Access to nursing notes by patients is decided using the strategy shown in the 'case study' below.
- Nursing notes are filed with medical records after discharge. Photocopies of the care plans, etc., can be given to the patient to hand to his or her community nurse where appropriate.

Case study

Comments on confidentiality with reference to access to notes by patients

1. The notes relate to *nursing* notes and not medical notes – specifically the content of care plans, assessment sheets and evaluation.
2. The basic assumption is that the patient has the right of access to the information with the right to comment on the content.
3. The primary nurse bears the responsibility for explaining *all* the implications to the patient of having access to notes, particularly in relation to matters of confidentiality, specifically:
   - An absolute guarantee of confidentiality cannot be made if notes are kept at the bedside (i.e. may be accessible for other patients, visitors or family to read without the patient's consent).
   - Potential problems can be minimised by following the suggested guidelines on access (see Figure 4.5).
   - Notes can be retained by the patient, either in the patient's locker or at the head of the bed, giving closer possession within the patient's personal space.
4. All nurses must be fully aware and skilled in completing nursing notes unambiguously and objectively as they may be asked to justify written phrases by the patient (and his family).
5. All nurses should read and fully understand the guidelines discussed in the UKCC advisory paper, specifically:

continued next page

continued

- The paragraph (clause nine) that reads:

  'Each registered nurse, midwife and health visitor is accountable for his or her practice, and in the exercise of professional accountability shall respect confidential information obtained in the course of professional practice and refrain from disclosing such information *without the consent* of the patient/client, or a person entitled to act on his/her behalf, except where disclosure is required by law or by order of a court or is necessary in the public interest'.

- In general, information on patients might be disclosed under a number of categories, among which is:

  '*With the consent of the patient/client*'

  Clearly this category does not constitute a breach of confidentiality, since consent implies that the patient's autonomy has been respected.

6. The patient's informed consent, once given, must be clearly documented/ dated and signed by the nurse responsible.

General points relating to patient's access to nursing notes

1. Patient's access to notes must be monitored continuously by the nurse in charge of the patient as part of the total programme of care.
2. Notes and care plans must be checked and reviewed daily by the primary nurse (or associate in his/her absence).
3. Contents of notes, when left at the bedside, must be reviewed with and explained to the patient by the nurse responsible for his/her care.
4. When in doubt, keep the nursing notes at the nurses' station until reviewed and discussed by the primary nurse with the sister/charge nurse.
5. The primary nurse should discuss 'sensitive' issues, i.e. dying or sexualising and the patient's degree of acceptance, with the sister or charge nurse prior to leaving the notes with the patient.
6. The patient's choice of access should be recorded in the nursing notes, particularly if consent has been given.
7. All patients' care plans are discussed with the patient by the nurse in charge of their care, regardless of their choice to retain the notes or not.
8. Patients' personal choices must be adhered to and respected at all times.
9. Any care plan or evaluation completed by a student nurse must be checked and countersigned by the registered nurse.
10. All potential primary nurses and practising primary nurses should improve and widen their knowledge basis in this area and must attend the appropriate training packages on the unit.
11. Patients are to be actively encouraged to read, comment upon, question the content of and write in their care plan if they wish to do so.

PATIENT ADMITTED – OFFERED CHOICE OF KEEPING NOTES AT BEDSIDE/NURSES' STATION – IMPLICATIONS EXPLAINED

If chooses to keep at bedside

a. Explain full implications and confidentiality issues

b. Record/date/sign when consent has been given in the nursing notes

↓

Keep nursing notes in a secure place with the patient, i.e. locker/bedhead

↓

Discuss contents of plans with patient at bedside

↓

a. Patient may write in evaluations if wishes

b. Check at regular intervals if patient is still happy about retaining notes

Wants to see notes but not keep them at bedside
(e.g. does not wish relatives to see them)

↓

Offer to let patient see notes on a daily basis or as requested by patient, e.g. at report-writing time

↓

a. Discuss contents of plans with patient at bedside

b. Retain notes at the nurses' station

↓

Patient may write in evaluation if he or she wishes

↓

Check at regular intervals for change of mind, if patient wishes to keep notes

Does not wish to keep notes

Explain that notes will be stored at the nurses' station

↓

a. Discuss contents of the plans with patient at the bedside

b. Retain notes at the nurses' station

↓

Patient may write in evaluation if he or she wishes

↓

Check at regular intervals to see if patient wishes to change mind (e.g. originally felt 'too ill' to bother and now improving)

Unable to make choice
(e.g. disorientated/unconscious)

↓

a. Explain that notes will be retained at the nurses' station where appropriate

b. Follow personal request of patient's close relatives (who have given all the details for assessment)

c. Primary nurse may choose to make decision for patient (if no relatives) and remain fully accountable/responsible for decision

d. Record/date/sign final decision in patient's notes

↓

When condition improves, discuss contents with patient and relatives at bedside

↓

Review with patient when able to make rational choice

Access to notes

Fig. 4.5   Guidelines on access to nursing notes by patients

11. How Do Student and Pupil Nurses Fit into the Scheme?

(Please refer also to question 8 above and to Chapter 2.)

The student nurse is not a qualified nurse and cannot act as a primary nurse. He or she may work as associate nurse, but should have 'off-duties' organised so that constant RGN supervision is maintained. The degree of involvement in care will vary according to the student's level of experience and ability. It is part of the role of the primary nurse to be a teacher/supporter of others. Indeed, primary nursing seems to facilitate this in line with the ENB (1987a) recommendations on the provision of 'mentoring' for students.

> The evaluations by students of their stay here (primary nursing ward) are rated really high. They have a much richer experience working with this ratio and a manageable group of patients. They seem to learn to manage the nurse–patient relationship better, get a more in-depth knowledge of the patient and his or her problems and are better able to develop and transfer their theoretical knowledge into practice.
>
> *Clinical teacher*

When the primary nurse or mentor is not on duty, the other primary nurses can ensure that students are helped and adequately supervised.

> For the first time, I felt I was learning to nurse here. I found it was better to get to know a few in depth rather than a lot superficially. I felt like part of the team and got to understand better about involvement with patients and how we can work 'with' them rather than 'at' them.
>
> *Student nurse*

Organising the workload with students remains a permanent problem while they are still allocated as part of the workforce. This is obviously not a problem specific to primary nursing and will remain until the position of students in the NHS is resolved.

12. Can Primary Nursing Work on Night Duty?

Yes. The roles need to be carefully worked through and joint meetings of staff arranged to identify working patterns. In general, it is very difficult for the night nurse to be a primary nurse because of the more restricted access to the multidisciplinary team, relatives or other carers. Again, it is important that the roles are clearly understood and valued. Being the associate nurse does not mean that the role is any less valuable than the primary nurse, nor does it mean that independent decisions about care cannot be made, or initial assessments and plans of care completed.

Much depends on the factors in each setting, e.g. whether internal rotation of day/night staff is feasible either for all or some of the staff, the number of part-time staff, skill mixes and so on. It is therefore difficult to lay down hard and fast rules; each setting is unique and must decide for itself the way forward. Certainly, where there is continuity of staff on nights in a unit and if, for example, the greater part of the patients' nursing problems are at night, there is no reason why the night nurse cannot act as the primary nurse.

The following case study illustrates some of these issues:

Case study

INTRODUCING PRIMARY NURSING TO NIGHT DUTY

As the night sister allocated to the ward, I was eager to learn as much as possible about primary nursing. This I did by reading papers and articles on the subject, including the ones produced by the staff on Ward X where primary nursing had already been introduced, discussions with other nursing staff and attending a conference on primary nursing.

For the day staff primary nursing was also a new innovation, so I felt this was the ideal opportunity for the day and night staff to improve their relationship with one another and break down the day/night barrier while improving the continuity of care given to the patient. I approached the introduction of primary nursing to night duty in the following way:

- • Many of the night staff I discussed primary nursing with were very pessimistic that it could be implemented successfully, while others were

continued next page

---

continued

totally opposed to the idea. A minority were enthusiastic and eager to gain further information on the topic; these were the staff I was hoping would be allocated to the ward!

- Because of the mixed reaction I received from the staff I decided it was the appropriate time to approach the night nurse manager to discuss the necessity of a stable night team, who were interested and motivated, to be allocated to the ward. The nurse manager was already aware of the impending arrival of primary nursing as I had ensured that she was informed of all up to date developments. She gave me her full support as far as possible but could not guarantee that the same team of nurses would always be allocated to the ward. This I was aware would be one of the greatest problems.
- I liaised closely with the day staff and attended meetings to discuss implementation of primary nursing and the role the night staff would play. The need for improved communication between day and night staff was paramount if we were to be successful.
- Many of the night staff found it difficult to attend meetings held by the day staff. I acted as their representative. The information I received was then related to other members of the night nursing team and we discussed ideas on the best way to approach primary nursing from a night point of view. In turn, key members of staff on days agreed to short spells of night duty, and meetings were held at night which day staff attended.
- I made a point of educating my colleagues about primary nursing. Literature was made available on the ward. I ensured I was available if the staff wished to discuss the subject. I also encouraged the staff to attend any courses or conferences relating to primary nursing.
- It was agreed with the day staff that the night nurse would on the whole take the role of associate nurse. In the event of the majority of problems a particular patient encountered occurring at night, then the RGN on night duty would take the role of primary nurse for the patient.
- The staff allocated to the ward at night often consists of an RGN, an SEN and a nursing auxiliary. Usually the RGN gives all of the report in hand-over time to the day staff. This changed as each trained nurse reported on his/her own patients.
- I also felt it important that the idea of the night staff carrying out a short spell on day duty, and vice versa, should be encouraged so that all problems would be appreciated by all members of the nursing staff. Communication between staff would be improved, leading to an improved 24-hour service for the patient.
- A white board was provided for ward use to enable the staff to specify which patients they were caring for. The night staff have been added to this

continued next page

continued

board and each was allocated a group of patients for whom they acted as associate nurse. The nurse acted as associate nurse for at least one spell of duty, i.e. three/four nights, if necessary, if the patient's length of stay was greater. (This was an acute ward – average length of stay for most patients was 7 days.)

- I found that the approach to primary nursing at night must be flexible and it will alter depending upon the ward situation and staffing levels. Each trained staff nurse acted as associate nurse for 12 patients, with the auxiliary nurse taking the role of aide or helper. The associate nurse carries out the care prescribed, writes the nursing notes and gives a report on her patients to the day staff, discussing any appropriate change of care with the primary nurse.

Night sister

There are therefore many implications for night staff in primary nursing. Remington (1989) notes: 'It would be a great mistake to see primary nursing as just the latest in a line of nursing fads that came in with a bang and go out with a whimper. Permanent night staff must be aware of what the concept entails and what the implications will be for them'.

The strength of the team, as suggested earlier, appears to be crucial in determining night staff involvement in, and commitment to, primary nursing. The issues are often emotive and revolve around feelings of status and being valued. Joint meetings, internal rotation, occasional exchange of shifts from days to nights and vice versa can all help to consolidate a team spirit, remove the sense of isolation that so often bedevils night nursing and help build up a collegiate relationship of mutual trust and understanding.

13. Can the Care Assistant be a Primary or Associate Nurse?

Primary nursing is clearly a role designated for the trained nurse, and, as has been suggested earlier, the associate may be a student nurse under certain circumstances. The care assistant/nursing auxiliary role is designed to assist the nurse to deliver care effectively (see Chapter 3). However, conflicts can arise if the care assistants are not fully included as a member of the team, and McFarlane and Castledine (1982) seem to suggest that they can be included as associates. They too have a vital role to play in promoting the 'primary nursing culture' and the sense of team spirit. They can, for example, still be involved in decisions which affect the unit and its policies, and particularly their own working practices. Working in teams with primary and associate nurses, they can retain supervised patient contact and continue to contribute through their help with, and observations on, patients and their care.

> As a nursing auxiliary on this unit I am as much a part of the team as everyone else. I take part in all the reporting sessions, and help the primary nurse with her patients. If I notice something about a patient, then I would tell her. I write things I notice in the nursing notes too.
>
> *Care assistant/nursing auxiliary, Elderly Care Unit*

It is essential that the degree of involvement and purpose in nursing is recognised, otherwise the nursing auxiliary/ care assistant can feel relegated to the role of mere kitchen cleaner and not an overall helper in care. In many settings nursing auxiliaries have been major care givers, and some may not relish the return to their true role. Sadly, this has occurred not because of a flaw in primary nursing, but because of failings in nursing as a whole. The nursing auxiliary should never have been led into a position where he or she is the assessor, planner, giver and evaluator of care, which has occurred in some settings. This is an abuse of the nursing auxiliary and an infringement of the patient's right to skilled nursing. As primary nursing develops, especially when the skill mix is changed, then the role of the true helper to the nurse and patient must emerge. The care assistant/nursing auxiliary should not be placed in a position where he or she replaces the trained nurse. Inevitably, some nursing auxiliaries can feel a sense of loss if required to adopt their true role, while others will feel more comfortable at having their role more clearly defined – and are not doing more than that which they are paid to do!

> Things were changing generally on the unit, not just primary nursing. Inevitably, some of the auxiliaries left because they didn't like being 'in charge' any more, but most fitted well into the new scheme of things. I felt sorry for those who felt unable to adapt. After all, it was our fault historically that had led them into a role for which they were not properly prepared or being rewarded. We encouraged quite a number to get into nurse training themselves – if they were that good they should be trained and paid for it.
>
> *Nurse manager*

14. Doesn't Primary Nursing Reinforce the Élitist Position of the Primary Nurse?

Previous sections of this chapter have emphasised the need for a strong team and collegiate spirit to promote primary nursing. Élites already exist in ward and community hierarchies. Primary nursing is not about élitism; it is about matching nurses to patients so that the patient gets the quality of care to which he or she has a right. Even the word 'primary' has a superior ring to it, being equated with the Latin word 'primus', meaning first. However, arguing over terminology would be a sterile debate. What matters more is the attitude of all nurses in the team, which recognises and values the roles of each other in meeting the patients' needs for care. The primary nurse is not necessarily the best person, but because of his or her added knowledge or skill should be the best equipped to solve the patient's nursing problems. Thus the primary nurse is not an élitist, but a thinking-doer, putting skills to the use of the patient and leading colleagues towards that central function.

15. What about the Medical and Other Staff?

Traditionally, in the hospital setting, when other disciplines have wanted information about a patient, they have tended to approach the ward sister or charge nurse. With autonomy and accountability devolved to each primary nurse, there is a risk of confusion, if not of hostility!

Responses in the studies seem to have been very varied. McFarlane and Castledine (1982) reported that 'our doctors just find it a little strange that, instead of consulting the ward sister about each patient, they had to relate more to the rest of the trained staff'. The 'visibility' notice suggested earlier appears to be as helpful to doctors as to nurses and patients. A programme of education of medical staff may be as important as that for the nurses. Responses may vary from (a) pleasure of many medical and other disciplines with the increased collaboration which occurs, to (b) others who have found primary nursing threatening because they are 'not in charge of nurses' (Hegyvary, 1982).

The experience of the Nursing Development Unit illustrates the following principal issues:

- Most members of the disciplines were, in practice, very supportive. They saw primary nursing as mirroring their own practice in some ways, and as having trained staff responsible for individual patients.
- The multidisciplinary team, as well as patients and relatives, have to be involved in the run-up to primary nursing. Explaining what it is all about and giving plenty of time for questions, involvement in unit meetings, trial periods, reassessments, and so on, will encourage co-operation.
- 'Selling' primary nursing to other disciplines was important in that they not only understood it, but could see advantages in it for them, i.e. they would know that a particular nurse had an in-depth knowledge of a particular patient, would be better able to assist them, and could be specifically identified (e.g. as opposed to 'passing the buck') when a problem of continuity of care arose.
- Being prepared for role conflicts, most specifically with some medical staff who have become accustomed to (and might prefer!) the ward sister or hand-maiden and fount of all knowledge about patients.
- Demonstrating that the quality of care has improved (e.g. from the results of quality assurance tests used).

- Demonstrating that other staff can have confidence in other nurses previously considered 'junior'.

Some of the doctors were hesitant at first, but it depends on how you manage the situation. We spent time explaining what it was all about beforehand. But in the end, there's nothing like experience for learning. Other professionals began to learn that they could trust the primary nurse simply because they experienced her knowledge and skills in relation to the patient. In some settings, colleagues adapted very quickly; in others it took longer to overcome the doubts. The ward sister/charge nurse's approach is particularly important in helping to wean the other disciplines away from complete dependence on him or her and in encouraging them to accept the new organisation. After a while, we were surprised how few problems we had in this area. We even had doctors coming back and telling us how surprised they were with the nurse's knowledge of the patient! The relationships began to change quite significantly.

Senior primary nurse/ward sister

Some problems can also occur for the sisters/charge nurses themselves (see earlier in the chapter) as they have to cope with the perception of other disciplines about the role. These perceptions of roles are discussed at length by Argyle (1978), who notes that conflict and 'role strain' may come from three main sources. It may arise between roles (for example, the working nurse who is also a wife and mother) or within a role (for example, the ward sister who must be both primary nurse and ward manager, yet the two may not always overlap easily). A third source is the conflict which occurs in the 'role set', the people nurses work with day to day who have different roles from the nurse and who have different perspectives on what nursing is. The ward sister/ charge nurse's role set, for example, would include patients, doctors, ward nursing colleagues, relatives and nursing officer.

To minimise such stresses and strains around the role of primary nurse, it is, therefore, essential that non-nursing colleagues are also prepared for what primary nursing is. That is not to say that nurses need, for example, to ask the doctors *if* they can start primary nursing. Rather, as colleagues in the multidisciplinary team, they should have the concept explained to them so that when the change begins they are less likely to meet resistance and hostility.

16. What Happens if the Patient is Transferred to a Non-primary Nursing Area?

Primary nurses can accompany the patient to that ward, or a nurse who will be allocated to that patient may pay a visit from his or her ward to meet the patient first. Primary nursing tends to raise expectations for patients, which may not be met in other areas where primary nursing is not being practised. Clearly, there has to be a very careful preparation of the patient beforehand if there is awareness that organisation of care may be different in another area; then the patient will find this less threatening.

> In some ways we've found this a positive thing. The expectation of patients has led the ward to look at their organisation of the care and use us for advice. Of course, there have been others who are just not ready for it and have shunned the very idea. It's important that the patient is aware that things may be a little different, and also not to imply that his care will be any the worse.
>
> *Primary nurse*

In the case of patients who are readmitted to a primary nursing area, it may well be that they return to the care of the previous primary nurse. Again, there should be no hard and fast rule about this. A degree of flexibility is needed to take account of factors such as the patient's and nurse's wishes, the length of the referral before readmission, the nature of the patient's renewed problems, and so on. The team need to make an early decision in the light of these factors, what is in the patient's best interests and, of course, what the patient's wishes are. In general, to promote continuity of care, it is desirable that the same patients have the same nurses where possible.

17. Perhaps the Patient Won't Like Me, or I Him, or Maybe all this Closeness Will Be too much of a Strain – How Does the Nurse Manage this Close Contact with Patients?

There is nothing in primary nursing that suggests that every nurse must like every patient and vice versa. However, it is the experience of the team contributing to this book that difficulties associated in working with some patients are greatly diminished. This could be due to a variety of factors, for example:

- The presence of a supportive team of colleagues as a precursor to and continuity requirement of primary nursing.
- The shift in emphasis of working with the patient and family as patients/companions.

'Difficult' patients are often labelled 'unpopular' (Stockwell, 1972) because they are demanding of the nurse's time and energy. Much of the basis for this lies in the patient's fears and insecurities, which, if the nurse is working freely with the patient as helper and information giver, can be greatly reduced.

Reports by the Health Service Ombudsman (1986, 1987, 1988) seem to indicate that the majority of patients' complaints centre around inadequate communication skills. In primary nursing, keeping the patient informed, explaining, teaching and taking account of his views are an integral part of his care. How many nurses have been told not to 'get involved' with patients? As has been suggested in the first chapters, primary nursing is all about being 'involved', so that the patient (and relatives too) is in a position to be an active participant in his own care .

At first we thought of dividing the patients up into 'our' groups. We agreed that, if any nurse was having conflict with a patient, then we could swap. In practice it just never happened. Some patients seemed less 'difficult', perhaps because they had developed more secure relationships with us.

Primary nurse

When I was working in the long stay areas, I thought this would really be a problem. So much so that, when we were 'starting out' we agreed to change our assignments after 3 months if necessary. We simply couldn't envisage wanting to stay with the same group of patients (or them with us). Of course, it just never happened! Something changes in the way you work with patients. The continuity of the relationship, and the rewards which come from that, seem to become more important than the change of scene.

Primary nurse

The assumption is often made that the nurse will need a change of patients. Primary nursing calls this into question. Of course, there is also the corollary that the patient may wish to make a change too! In general, both circumstances should be extremely rare. The writers have all been primary nurses where many thousands of patients have passed through our care. Although the proviso was made that nurse and patient could change assignments, this happened only once in 5 years. (In this instance, a patient refused to have any contact with a particular nurse. The ward then discussed the problem, and the nurse himself felt he should be reassigned because of the risk of the added stress to the patient.)

The approach to assignment needs to remain open and flexible, as follows:

- There should be no hard and fast rule about length of assignment. Experience has shown that, despite fears to the contrary, the nurses themselves will not, ultimately, put a time limit on it.
- Added stress for the nurse can be produced when the patient is more demanding, i.e. in need of more physical or psychological attention from her, i.e. the patient's dependency level is greater. Thus, primary nurses' caseloads should not be fixed. Some nurses might have seven patients, others three, in the same unit. The level needs to be determined by the needs of patients. Conflicts with patients may often arise because the nurse is not fulfilling her role with all patients because of an over-stretched caseload.

● While the primary nurse is accountable for the patient's care over 24 hours, it does not mean that she is 'on call' 24 hours a day! The associate nurse is an accountable trained nurse too and should not normally need to seek help from the primary nurse outside normal working hours. When help is needed, there will normally be other primary/senior nurses available to assist. However, if the primary nurse wishes to be involved, then there is no reason why this should not be so.

> Being called up at home is an extremely rare occurrence. It happened a few times on this ward in the past few years. It might be because the primary nurse has overlooked something important and the associate nurse needs to call her to check. However, it's more likely that the primary nurse herself has asked to be called. I can think of one instance when a patient, with no known relatives, was dying. The primary nurse asked to be called in if anything happened during the night.
>
> *Senior primary nurse/ward sister*

● Managing the nurse–patient relationship in nursing requires a supportive team of colleagues in any circumstances. This is no less so in primary nursing. Flexibility with rules in relation to workload and length of assignment is essential. In practice, changing nurses and patients will be a rare event. A climate that allows nurses to express their feelings about patients is also needed – which does not criticise the nurse who becomes upset because a patient dies, or censure her because she is having difficulty managing a patient's problems. If close contact is more demanding of nurses, this cannot be countenanced without the right climate to support the nurses.

● *Patient contact hours.* Most authors agree that the relationship between nurse and patient is easier to develop where the patient is in for a longer stay. What about the short term? Manthey (1980) has this to say:

'Since the patient will be receiving some nursing during his short stay, I see no reason why he should not know the name of the nurse responsible for that care. Someone will be making some kind of decisions'.

She goes on to argue that:

'It may not be necessary to have a nursing care plan for the short-term patient, but primary nursing is visible responsibility for decision making, not the existence of elaborate care plans'.

In addition, staff who work part time or as 'bank nurses' are affected by their limitations of contact hours with the patient. Whether or not the part-time nurse is a primary nurse will depend upon the number of hours worked and the length of stay of the patient.

● Primary nursing is also not necessarily synonymous with documentation/care planning. Many nurses might ask how they can be expected to primary nurse when they seem to have little time as it is to plan care! Of course, the two are related, but quite separate. Manthey (1988) notes succinctly:

'Primary nursing is not synonymous with care plans! Primary nursing requires that each patient know the name of his or her primary nurse. Primary nursing also requires that each primary nurse be responsible for giving and co-ordinating whatever care the patient receives during the hospital stay. With short-term patients, primary nurses learn to perform short-term, realistic assessments and set short-term, realistic goals. Whether care plans are written is a separate issue of communication and/or documentation'.

Thus, whether it be in operating theatres or casualty department, the principles of primary nursing can still apply. A named nurse, known to the patient, can be allocated to care for him, no matter how short the time. In fact it might be argued that in high-activity areas (often associated with a great deal of threat to the patients), having a reassuring person to whom the patient can relate is even more essential. For example:

(i) The anaesthetic nurse might visit the patient in the surgical ward prior to operation.
(ii) Surgical nurses working on day case wards work

flexible hours to be present during the whole of the allocated patient's stay.

(iii) The nurse in casualty carries out the care for 'her' patients while they are in the department.

18. Do Tasks Disappear?

Not necessarily. What might be called 'housekeeping' duties are clearly the role of the care assistant, to enable the trained nurse to get on with the job of nursing. At other times, better use might be made of the ward clerk or secretarial role. Functions such as managing the ward budget, re-ordering stores, planning off-duties, etc., can either be delegated to ward clerks (in some settings these have become ward 'managers' or 'co-ordinators') or dispersed in rotation among the staff.

In general, everybody seems to hate doing the non-nursing jobs like checking the linen supplies or planning the off-duty. We made sure that some jobs were clearly the work of the assistants; we focused on the nursing. The assistants would then also help us with things that needed two persons (e.g. lifting) as well as helping each other.

We also delegated things like off-duty planning, ordering stores, etc., among ourselves, e.g. one nurse would do the off-duties for a month, another the stores checking, and so on. It also meant that each member of staff had some experience in these things.

Senior primary nurse/charge nurse

Sometimes it seems more difficult to escape the tasks because they are bound up in hospital procedure and policy books.

Medicines used to be carried out by a strict two-person procedure. Eventually, we obtained a new medicine trolley with individual dispensers. Each patient's medicines were contained in a separate box, topped up by the pharmacist each day. The primary nurse could simply take medicines from the box labelled

continued next page

continued _____

for each patient without having to take the whole trolley. That way each primary or associate nurse saw to it that 'their' patients got their medicines. We managed to get rid of the 'round'.

Primary nurse

Activities that are focused on the patient are carried out by the primary/associate nurse for that patient. Dividing patients up into neatly packaged procedures (the 'temps', the 'BPs', the 'dressings') is incompatible with primary nursing.

19. What about Primary Nursing in the Community?

The principles of primary nursing (see Chapters 1 and 2) are universal. Manthey (1988) describes the concept of 'my nurse: my neighbour'. The question is an organisational one. The primary (community) nurse has a case load of patients and addresses herself to the patients' nursing needs as a whole.

Each nurse in the clinic took his or her own case load of patients. Sometimes we worked flexi hours if, say, the patient required some aspect of care in the evening. Otherwise, an associate nurse would go in, but the overall planning and co-ordination of care remain with the primary nurse.

Primary nurse in community care

In many respects, community nursing has tended to retain many elements of Nightingale's 'case method' approach. However, community based care runs an equal risk of being fragmented to that of hospital based care. However, it is true that much of the writing on primary nursing has tended to focus on the hospital setting. Perhaps this is not surprising in view of the overwhelming tendency of hospitals to produce regimented patterns of care, which negates the personal needs of individual patients. Primary nursing represents the effort to reverse that trend.

It may be that the patient does not require nursing in the community. The hospital primary nurse may hand the patient over to another 'key worker', e.g. domiciliary physiotherapist or social worker, who will then take over meeting the patient's principal need. In some circumstances, where no particular help is needed at home, primary nurses in hospital might retain their contact with the patient.

> Sometimes we found that patients going home were not in need of any particular help. But we made it known that we were available if advice was needed. Occasionally patients will ring up and ask to speak to their primary nurse if a problem crops up and the patient is not sure who to approach. We can either deal with it or put them in touch with the appropriate person.
>
> *Primary nurse*

20. How Do you Introduce Primary Nursing?

Planning the change has been emphasised in the earlier chapters. Having read some of the questions, the reader might well be induced to ask, 'Well, how do *I* do it?' The following is a progress report which draws together some of these strands:

How I Implemented Primary Nursing

The Early Stages

- I developed my self-knowledge and self-awareness as a ward sister and found a 'vision'. I researched everything on primary nursing and examined the beliefs and the present practice on the ward.
- I compared our philosophy and practice with that of primary nursing.
- I educated myself by reading articles given to me by other colleagues and visited other staff who were already implementing primary nursing.
- Articles about the topic were gathered from nursing journals, books, etc.

- We talked with colleagues in other wards and in other hospitals to gain as much information as possible.
- I reviewed our understanding of the philosophy of primary nursing to make sure that I had a clear picture of what my goals were (i.e. by exchanging views with more senior and experienced colleagues, teachers, etc.).
- Primary nursing conferences and study days were attended.
- I sought advice and guidance from other nurses, especially from those who had already implemented primary nursing and who had more information and experience.
- The pitfalls, disadvantages and obstacles I was likely to encounter were identified and taken into consideration in the clinical area of a busy acute medical ward.

The Vision

- Once I felt fully confident and secure, and had a strong, clear picture of my goal, I felt that I had to communicate this to the rest of my ward staff. They too had to share the same vision and philosophy and strong motivation with regard to primary nursing for it to be successfully implemented on the ward. Everyone from nursing auxiliary to staff nurse had to think and progress in the same direction.

    In order to increase the staff's motivation, eagerness and willingness, and to develop and share the same beliefs, I spent time with the following aspects:

    (i) The simplicity of primary nursing philosophy was discussed, i.e. the roles of a primary nurse, associate nurse and care assistant were defined. We planned ways that these roles could be co-ordinated together in a team to promote individualised nursing care.
    (ii) Time was taken at every opportunity to chat to staff at breaks, while making beds and during simple nursing procedures, stressing the ways in which the new philosophy (primary nursing) could be applied practically.
    (iii) Slowly, once the term 'primary nursing' was fami-

liar on the ward to day and night staff and to doctors, etc., we had formal talks on the ward. Staff from other primary nursing wards were invited to come and talk to us about 'how they did it'. Each nurse on the ward participated in discussion and questioning.

(iv) We established regular ward meetings after 8.30 p.m. in order that night staff could be present.

(v) Regular meetings were held with trained nurses to explore the importance of the accountability and responsibility of primary nurses and associate nurses.

(vi) Enrolled nurses were given the choice of being primary nurses after all the responsibilities involved were explained. They all declined and were quite happy to become associate nurses.

(vii) The tutorial staff and others sought to explain to staff the importance of accountability and responsibility and the type of vocabulary and documentation to which we would have to adapt when keeping care plans at the patient's bedside. The importance of confidentiality was discussed.

(viii) The nursing officer was involved in our plans to implement primary nursing as we needed the support and understanding of management. Close liaison with the nursing officer, in terms of the problems encountered, e.g. the off-duty rota, lack of trained staff, etc., was vital.

(ix) In order to stimulate staff, study days were arranged at other hospitals for members of staff to attend in order to bring back fresh ideas and information. It was important to keep them interested and involved in preparation.

(x) I sought to maintain communication with all members of staff, especially night staff.

Separate meetings were held with nursing auxiliaries, enrolled nurses and registered general nurses together to gain their ideas and views and to listen to their anxieties.

(xi) Each member of staff was interviewed and asked

personally if he or she felt happy about working on a ward practising primary nursing. Advantages were highlighted in order to be positive and encouraging. Particular attention was paid to those who were unsure, not interested or lacking in knowledge.

(xii) The importance of all grades of staff was reinforced, and the significant role of associate nurse, care assistant and primary nurse were clearly defined.

Creating a Primary Nursing Climate

Once I felt that the staff had a thorough understanding and positive view of primary nursing, I began to choose teams:

> 24 patients   4 RGNs   4 ENs   4 NAs
>   = 6 patients each

- Originally, groups were organised by the ward staff, but as the skill mix is extremely important, some teams were changed to prevent personality clashes or conflicts, to avoid other management problems and to balance expertise.
- The off-duty rota was done by me at first in order to make sure that there was always a primary nurse working opposite to an associate nurse, and that care was being maintained by the same team.
- The staff had to be involved in the off-duty planning with the rule that each was 'covered' by the other. Requests had to be kept to a minimum as the priority was to ensure that each group of patients always had their primary or associate nurse on duty.
- Marker boards were placed on the ward, where, weekly, each trained nurse was responsible for writing about an aspect of primary nursing. The comment was left on the ward for another week in order that everyone could read it. The response was very good as each member was actively involved, and they enjoyed the frequent turnover of fresh information.
- Visitors were encouraged to come to the ward and exchange ideas with staff.

- Books and leaflets were available for everyone to read.

The Final Preparation

- Doctors were involved at the regular ward sessions. Each primary nurse became responsible for the ward round of her own group of patients (four bays of six) and for their admission and discharge programme. There was a deliberate ploy to avoid sisters doing a full ward round and to encourage them to refer to the appropriate primary nurses. Other staff, such as the ward clerk, also had to be made aware that a telephone call, visitor or any other patient problem should be referred to the appropriate primary or associate nurse. Referring everything through the ward sister (the usual way of doing things) is incompatible with primary nursing.
- Photographs of the nurses accompanied the nurse's name at the bedside.
- The primary nurses, associate nurses and care assistants were identified to each patient. Name badges were supplied which included the nurse's role, e.g. senior primary nurse/ward co-ordinator.

NB   It was very important for me to hand over the authority and to take a step back and allow the staff to make the final decisions. The sister role changed drastically to that of support, teaching and guidance. The staff had to understand this too. I had to create a new role. Asking the primary nurse to arrange ambulances and to work with the consultant was a conscious effort on my part, and I had to concentrate on staff development and see myself as a resource. I tried to help, advise and support every member of staff, including the night staff, who were involved in all the new activities. I had regular meetings with them.

Senior primary nurse/ward sister

Finally

Don't be too firm about the time schedule – take the plunge and do it!

Many questions arise over primary nursing, and, hopefully, some of these will have been answered in the preceding pages, However, there is an old adage, as the Joni Mitchell quote at the beginning of this chapter suggests, that there is no education like experience. Having grasped the vision, it is up to each nurse and each team of nurses to pursue it in their own way.

CHAPTER 5

Helping it to Happen – the Roles of Manager and Educator

*Prometheus, by his free will, undertook and carried
out his plan, though he knew very well the consequences of his action. He had other alternatives, but
he chose the nobler one and committed himself to his
decision, which was to help men do better by making
them masters of their minds.*

Vassiliki Lanara
Heroism as a Nursing Value

In previous chapters, it has often been noted how the change
to primary nursing must come from nurses themselves.
However, it has also been stressed that it cannot be left to
the clinical nurses alone. They too have needs, most
importantly for that supportive climate that enables them to
'get on with it'. This chapter explores some of the characteristics of the support which primary nursing needs, and how
the manager and educator can contribute.

THE MANAGER'S ROLE

How can the manager facilitate primary nursing? The
following case study from a nurse manager illustrates many
of the principal elements of the manager's role:

First and foremost, I had to avoid the feeling among the staff that I wanted to push it (primary nursing) through. Indeed I had many uncertainties myself. How much would it cost me? Would care get better? Would the staff be happier? So I needed to think through and get information on a lot of those issues myself first. I saw my role as waiting for each ward to be ready for primary nursing, then moving in with the support when they needed it.

To be brief, some of the points of my input included the following:

- Giving time for the staff to develop at their own pace.
- Helping the staff to review the skill mix so that it would be appropriate to primary nursing. For example, my unit was heavily staffed with nursing auxiliaries – almost 80%; over time as they left I replaced them with trained staff. Currently this is now 65% trained staff – quite an about-turn, and I'm aiming for 80%. Of course there are fewer people about, but the qualities and qualifications of the staff are that much greater. By and large, I found that you could replace every 10 auxiliaries who left with about 6 trained staff for about the same cost.
- Providing resources, e.g. help with redesigning stationery, photographs, notice boards, etc., and all the peripheral things that nurses seem to need as adjuncts to primary nursing.
- Keeping the staff levels as stable as possible, including night duty, and avoiding borrowing of staff unless absolutely essential.
- Keeping an 'open door' policy so that staff could see me when needed. Also, 'walking the patch'! – being seen in the clinical areas, helping when necessary, listening to staff and their problems and involving them in decisions. A non-autocratic approach is essential.
- Helping to co-ordinate meetings of the unit's staff.
- Using praise and encouragement to reinforce the staff in their efforts, making a point of complimenting people on good work and letting them know when a positive comment or report has been made.
- Enabling the staff to participate in further development

courses, working with educators and facilitating 'networking'.

- Offering advice and counselling based on my experience, and acting as an outside 'problem solver' to be used by the ward staff.
- Appraising the staff and guiding their individual development and wishes.
- Monitoring sickness and absenteeism levels, and keeping an eye open for signs of stress arising.
- Monitoring the quality of care; as care was clearly improving, according to our quality assurance results, making sure the staff knew the results.
- Involving the ward sister/charge nurse in recruitment/interviewing so that nurses chosen are more likely to fit in with the team and share similar values.
- Supporting all the staff, but the sister/charge nurse in particular, for it is they who can feel most stressed as they relinquish power and delegate responsibilities.
- Relinquishing power myself! – letting the staff have more direct control over their budgets, skill mixes, off-duties, etc.
- Being a master juggler of the staffing establishment and my budget! Primary nursing had to be included amongst my overall objectives.
- Participating in 'selling' primary nursing to other managers and members of the multidisciplinary team, and at a wider level in the health authority, so that it becomes official policy.
- Accepting myself that I must adapt to a raised level of assertiveness and self-awareness among the staff.
- Being wary of giving the staff conflicting signals, i.e. it's no good telling the staff, 'OK, get on with it, be autonomous', and at the same time expecting them to obey my orders without question. To a greater or lesser degree, depending on his existing style, the manager in primary nursing has to undergo changes too. You have to be prepared to explain your actions and help the staff to understand your own role so they don't feel that you are interfering with or controlling them.
- Stepping in with support when needed, even when they

have made mistakes. Be realistic about primary nursing; it won't make everything perfect overnight.

There are many ways in which the manager can support primary nurses, but the above would be my 'top twenty' to start the ball rolling, and keep it going.

Just as the ward sister or charge nurse sets the style or climate of a ward, so the nurse manager can set the climate for a whole unit. Managers, too, need to be risk-taking, creative people in order to foster such values among their staff.

Price Waterhouse (1988) and McLure et al (1983) both indicated that the manager has a key role in promoting job satisfaction for staff. In so doing, he or she does much to resolve recruitment and retention problems. Involving the staff in decision-making, listening to the difficulties and helping to resolve problems are crucial elements in creating a satisfactory climate for the staff. At the same time, if primary nursing puts nurses in a position to nurse in the way they would like (inability to do this is a strong dissatisfaction to nurses – Price Waterhouse, 1988), another opportunity to enhance staff recruitment and retention arises.

JOB DESCRIPTIONS

These can be completely redesigned on the lines of primary nursing. Alternatively, a simple modification outlining the role occupied could be added in agreement with the staff. Clinical grading is another (thorny) issue in relation to this. Depending on the specific requirements of the role, the primary nurse must be allocated at least E/F grade, while C/D would seem most appropriate to the associate nurse. The manager has to make decisions on these issues at each stage, and in particular establish the appropriate mix of skills and grades with the ward team (see Appendix).

The creation of a stable, satisfied workforce should be the key goal of any nurse manager. It is no less essential in primary nursing.

EDUCATIONAL SUPPORT

The demands made of the role of the primary nurse require a programme of continuous education. This, it might be argued, should be the case for nurses anyway. However, there are additional and immediate aspects in primary nursing. The newly qualified nurse is rarely equipped to be launched ready-made into primary nursing. Whether, in the light of Project 2000, this situation will change remains to be seen, as it will, in any case, take many years for the effects of a new preparation of nurses to work through the system.

> The appropriate role for the newly qualified nurse should be that of associate nurse. In this role she can develop her skills, learning particularly from her primary nurse colleagues. On our unit we find that at least 6 months preparation is essential before the nurse is ready to take on her own permanent caseload.
>
> *Clinical nurse specialist*

Of course, each nurse has her own professional responsibility to keep up to date. However, it is the role of the manager in primary nursing to enable the staff to get the further development they need, and the role of the educator to provide it. Particular areas, of course, are the needs to enhance communication and problem-solving skills, as well as to deepen the understanding of the therapeutic value of nursing. Nurses also need to become aware of the consequences of greater autonomy and accountability and to explore the value system that they are using that underpins their day-to-day practice:

> Because of the need to heighten awareness of primary nursing issues among the staff, we designed a 2-week course, provided on site for them, and led by the clinical specialist, covering the following main topics.
>
> **The therapeutic basis of nursing**
>
> A part-time course for registered and enrolled nurses providing information and updating on current issues in clinical nursing:
>
> *continued next page*

continued

1. The value of nursing, its essence and actions in helping and healing.
   Partnership and companionship.
   Advocacy.
2. Nursing models – what they are and their importance to practice.
   Creative thinking in nursing.
3. The nursing process – putting the model into action through problem solving.
   Different approaches.
   Problems with care plans.
4. Primary nursing.
   Organising care to promote patient-centred practice.
   Setting up primary nursing.
5. Primary nursing II – primary nursing in practice.
6. Primary nursing III – evaluation and accountability.
7. Changing nursing – the application of change theory to nursing practice; developing the skills of being a change agent.
8. Therapeutic nursing; 'hands on' care.
   The nurse's helping role.
   Complementary therapies – their relevance to nursing.

Clinical nurse specialist

The sample course outlined above was subsequently developed and considerably expanded. It may well form the basis of a formal postgraduate course on the subject. It is worth noting that much of the development of nurses in primary nursing focuses on developing their expressive skills – those related to communicating with, teaching and comforting patients. Some of the complementary therapies (e.g. reflexology, therapeutic touch, therapeutic massage and aromatherapy) have also been useful in enhancing the nurse's abilities in 'touching' patients and contributing to the overall notion of nursing as a healing or therapeutic act.

We set up a 'complementary therapies group', invited guest speakers each month and learned to practise various therapies with each other. We found them helpful in improving our awareness, for example, of the importance of touch and our abilities to do it more effectively.

Senior primary nurse

Courses and workshops, however, should not only concentrate on content, but also on method. Experiential techniques, role play, and so on, are all essential to develop greater awareness and assertiveness among nurses, and to enhance their communication skills.

It is also important that those nurses developing primary nursing have a chance to meet with others doing likewise (i.e. 'networking'). Both managers and educators can facilitate this at local, regional and national level.

> We organised 'primary nursing peer support group' meetings on the unit. These were a great source of getting together, reinforcing ideas, sharing problems and getting mutual support. The manager also provided funding so that some of us could attend the primary nursing network meetings organised by the King's Fund, both in London and regionally.
>
> *Primary nurse*

It is particularly important that possibilities of providing 'on-site' education are explored, so that it appears relevant to the staff's day-to-day practice. Some of the following points need to be considered:

- Is a support team or teacher available to work with the staff in the clinical setting, e.g. the nurse manager, clinical teacher or tutor, or clinical nurse specialist?
- Part-time as well as full-time courses need to be provided. Some staff may wish to attend in their own time, otherwise the manager needs to support 'time off' as far as possible.
- Development should be available to all staff. This includes untrained staff as well. The role of the care assistant, for example, can be woven into courses for nursing auxiliaries.
- Staff development opportunities also need to include aspects of nursing management. Some primary nurses need to evolve into the general managers and senior nurse managers of the future.
- Multidisciplinary workshops, etc., may also be needed to raise awareness of primary nursing among colleagues.

- Staff from the school of nursing can assist by supporting the staff in the clinical area by providing facilities in the school for nurses for workshops and seminars, and by organising speakers and workshop leaders.
- The student nurse should be prepared in advance about primary nursing, particularly in preparation for working in areas where primary nursing is practised.
- Access to literature, library resources, etc., is essential either in the school of nursing or in the clinical area, and preferably in both.
- Special arrangements for access to courses, literature, etc., should be made available for night staff.
- Distance learning packages can be designed for staff who may have difficulty in getting access to formal courses (especially night staff and part-time staff).
- Staff development meetings can be held to enable the staff to identify their own learning needs. These can also emerge at regular career counselling sessions. It might be helpful if, in any primary nursing unit, at least one senior nurse, clinical specialist or consultant nurse is delegated this function.

It wasn't just a question of gaining knowledge. We found that primary nurses also needed to become more aware of themselves, of their communication skills, and of their potential as 'change agents'. We devised an intensive 'survival skills course', covering all these kinds of topics, and made considerable use of role play, group work and experiential techniques to heighten awareness and develop skills and coping strategies.

Consultant nurse

Whether staff development is provided on or off site will largely depend upon the resources and personnel available. Local colleges and universities can be helpful where there are limitations in the health authority. Inevitably, where funding resources are limited, some staff might have to meet costs themselves. However, in some settings, staff have been able to enhance their resources by various fund-raising techniques (Purdy et al, 1988).

Kramer (1974) has argued that the preparation of nurses tends to produce a variety of different types of nurses, among them the 'rutters' (nurses who simply get along with their work and do not challenge the established order of nursing) and the 'bicultural troublemakers' (nurses who learn to survive within the organisation, yet become a force for change). Primary nursing, it seems, requires many more of the latter – nurses who can be creative, knowledgeable doers (Pearson and Vaughan, 1986). Producing more nurses of this calibre requires managers and educators to help them, even with the knowledge that life with more 'trouble-makers' may be less smooth! It needs a shift in the service sector (to accept that it has a duty to develop its staff, when it is not already doing so). The education of nurses cannot be abrogated entirely to the school of nursing.

At the same time, the teachers of nurses themselves might have to examine their practices. There is a need to accept the challenge of change (ENB, 1987b), to become active change agents themselves. The primary nurse is in the business of changing nursing and changing people's lives on a day-to-day basis. This cannot be done without the kind of management and educational support described in this chapter.

CHAPTER 6

Review and Conclusion

Make voyages! – Attempt them!
– There's nothing else

Tennessee Williams
Camino Real

So far, the authors have sought to describe what primary nursing is, and what important features underpin it. Issues related to day-to-day operation of primary nursing have been discussed to show how it might work in a variety of settings. Clearly, from the preceding chapters the authors have considerable enthusiasm for and commitment to primary nursing; the experiences of them and their patients suggest that there are many positive attributes which far outweigh any difficulties encountered.

DOES IT WORK?

Evidence for or against primary nursing is very varied. Much has been written about it, but often from an anecdotal and subjective standpoint. Research, where it has been conducted, is alleged to have many flaws. Young et al (1981) and Giovanetti (1987) have conducted extensive surveys of published research and other papers on primary nursing. The majority of the evidence on this basis is undoubtedly in favour of primary nursing for the following reasons:

- The patient feels more secure and satisfied as the nurse–patient relationship develops.
- The developing relationship increases job satisfaction for nurses.
- Nurses recognise that they can make judgments acceptable both to themselves and to patients.
- Nurses gain a clearer definition of their role in the multidisciplinary team.
- A sense of involvement with patient and family is gained by the nurse, with a resulting heightened sense of responsibility for care.
- Students' and trained nursing staff's sense of learning increases.
- Nurses feel more secure in professional function.
- Continuity of care is greater; there are fewer errors and patient complaints.
- Nurses develop their skills as teachers, both with patients and colleagues.
- Patient care is more likely to be given as planned if the person planning care is also the care giver.
- Some reports suggest that, overall, the quality of care is improved, especially in relation to attention to patients' families, patient teaching and discharge planning.
- Use of equipment and of stores and commodities is improved.
- Fewer complaints and more patient contact produces more trusting nurse–patient relationships.
- Clarification and resolution of patients' problems is made easier through more awareness of the patient's needs.
- Group cohesion among nurses improves (although some nurses have reported increased competitiveness).
- Patient care becomes easier and more efficient (although some nurses have suggested that the close personal contact may make nursing care more strenuous and exhausting).
- Contact and understanding with medical staff increases (although some doctors dislike not having 'sister' in overall control).
- Overall costs are reduced, especially in relation to more efficient use of resources and deployment of staff.

- Methods of documenting care improve.
- Nurses are better able to identify the 'gaps' in their knowledge and skill and identify their own learning needs.

The effects on patients and relatives of the introduction of primary nursing

I recently completed a project entitled 'The Primary Nursing Approach' as part of the ENB 941 course (Care of Elderly People). To help me to summarise and evaluate the effects of the introduction of primary nursing on a rehabilitation/ continuing care ward, I carried out a small-scale survey on the effects of primary nursing on 15 patients and their relatives.

I found that all patients and relatives were in favour of primary nursing. Results suggested that relatives understood the role of the primary nurse, and an overall comment was that they felt this aspect of giving care was a better way of nursing their relatives.

Comments from the patients were very rewarding, such as:

'It's like being looked after by my own family', 'I like having my nurse looking after me – I always look out for her because I know she looks after me and knows me better than anyone else'.

From the relatives' point of view the results were summarised as the following:

'Questions can be asked directly to the primary nurse who knows her patient inside out, and answers are obtained almost immediately, so fears and anxieties are allayed and confidence is assured'.

'It's advantageous to be able to speak to the same person caring for my relatives all the time – if I have a problem or am worried about something, I can talk to the primary nurse or associate nurse and problems are sorted out much more quickly'.

Individual comments from the patients included the following:

'It's nice to have the same person looking after me – getting me up in the morning and putting me to bed at night'.

'You get used to your own special nurse and she gets used to you too – she understands my problems better than anyone else'.

'I love my primary nurse'.

Results from the relatives' questionnaire showed that they were all in favour of primary nursing and felt that their relatives received a better quality of care on the primary nursing ward when compared to the acute ward from which their relative had been transferred, which practised conventional patient allocation/ team nursing.

continued next page

continued

Relatives' comments included the following:

'The patients seem to respond better towards their own special nurse – it's good to be able to discuss their care with the same people all the time – I can think of no disadvantages'.

'Questions can be asked and answered so much more quickly and confidence is assured at all times – there can only be advantages for this way of nursing patients'.

The summary reinforced our view that primary nursing can be seen as not only more rewarding and fulfilling for the practising primary nurse giving the care required, but also as a more satisfying, therapeutic and reassuring way of receiving care from the patient's point of view.

Primary nurse

Whether it be larger scale projects such as those of Marram (1976), Shukla (1983) or Giovanetti (1987), or smaller scale ones such as that cited in the case study above (Wills, 1988), there seems to be a large body of evidence expressing positive views of primary nursing.

With such an enormous range of alleged benefits, it is little wonder that a primary nursing 'bandwagon' got under way (Wright, 1988) in the UK. Beset by many troubles, it seems that the search by nurses to find their panacea is not a new phenomenon. Throughout nursing history, innovations have been taken up with wild enthusiasm and applied with great energy, but with little consideration for the evidence of real or imagined benefits or disadvantages. Is primary nursing falling into this trap?

Certainly, if primary nursing were to go ahead solely on the basis of uncontrovertible evidence, it would never have happened at all.

Giovanetti (1987), for example, cites many methodological inconsistencies in the research she surveyed: lack of definition of primary nursing, doubts about whether like is compared with like, size of samples, and so on. MacDonald (1988) notes how much of the available literature is of North American origin and thereby questions its applicability to the UK nursing culture and organisation of health care. Arguments ensue as to whether it is cheaper or more expensive to implement primary nursing. Shukla (1983) found evidence for increased staffing costs, while Binnies's (1987) work suggests these may be less. Variables, then, have to be considered, e.g. skill mix and experience of staff, and grades of pay may all cloud the issue.

Giovanetti (1987) also notes how 'calling a nurse a primary nurse and assuring continuity of patient assignment, for example, did not automatically result in increased authority, responsibility and accountability'. Manthey (1980), meanwhile, argues that merely organising primary nursing is of itself no guarantee of improved quality of care, although it should put nurses in a position where they are empowered to do better: 'Many people have mistakenly equated the concept of a system of care delivery with the concept of quality of care. The quality of nursing service in primary nursing can be good or bad, comprehensive or incomplete, co-ordinated or spasmodic, individualised or standardised, creative or routine'.

Throughout this text it has been argued that it is insufficient simply to reorganise groups of nurses and their skill mix. It is necessary also to examine the *values and attitudes* that underpin their practice and the *knowledge and skill* with which they practise. These factors are as crucial to primary nursing, and as inseparable from it, as the way in which nurses are deployed.

A fundamental principle of primary nursing is that, in reorganising nurses, there is a concurrent planned approach to question, develop and, where necessary, change the whole philosophy and practice of nurses and their care. The commitment to primary nursing is nothing less than this.

Bowers (1989) succinctly summarises and posits a number of other issues in relation to primary nursing. It may merely be a symptom of the desire for more professional status by nurses and part of a long history of attempts by nurses to wean themselves away from the control of others, notably doctors and latterly general managers. He raises questions about autonomy and accountability – how can nurses exercise these when others are constantly telling them what to do? How can they be responsible for the quality of care when so much of it (e.g. the provision of resources) is dependent on others? How far does primary nursing represent a desire by managers to control costs and nurses? (Managers would find it easier to identify an individual accountable nurse.) Meanwhile, primary nursing might put at risk the cohesiveness of the ward team or uncover 'conflicts between doctors and nurses' (Bowers, 1989).

Bowers further argues that there is a political dimension in the UK to the adoption of primary nursing:

> 'The rise of Thatcherism and the new right is having an impact on nursing in the UK. Large public bureaucracies are now believed to be inefficient. Structural changes are being made in order to make the system appear more efficient. Primary nursing fits hand in glove with these notions' (Bowers, 1989).

In the rush towards primary nursing, a bandwagon has been set in motion that tends to swamp the many doubts around it. As has been argued in earlier chapters, the traditional ward team may be less than the cohesive unit it is imagined to be, and it is the experience of all the contributors that team spirit tends to increase, not diminish, with primary nursing. Issues of accountability and autonomy have produced gross dissatisfaction with care, from both nurses and patients, in the past. Primary nursing is a manifestation of the effort to resolve these dilemmas. Meanwhile, the 'doctor–nurse game' (Stein, 1978), based on the accepted power structure between the two, leaves much to be desired.

'The doctor–nurse game' describes the relationship between doctor and nurse as an elaborately ritualised façade. In this way, nurses are able to manipulate the doctor's decision without overtly undermining his status or authority. Each partner has to be acutely sensitive to the non-verbal and cryptic cues given by the other. Each learns the game through a long process of socialisation as each gains experience in their respective fields. Stein says:

> 'The nurse is to be bold, have initiative and be responsible for making significant recommendations, while at the same time she must appear passive. This must be done in such a manner as to make her recommendations appear to be initiated by the physician'.

Thus, open disagreement between doctor and nurse is to be avoided at all costs and the nurse can communicate her recommendations without appearing to make a recommendation statement.

This strategy appears to help both doctor and nurse defuse what could otherwise be a very conflict-ridden area of their work. However, this restricts an honest dialogue and may stifle initiative. Nursing knowledge and skill is cloaked, and appreciation of its true value may be lost. It is not clear how the end product of this social 'pas-de-deux' between doctor and nurse benefits the patient. If primary nursing upsets the status quo between doctors, nurses and other disciplines, perhaps this is long overdue. Where a truly collegiate relationship already exists, primary nursing will probably enhance, not diminish, relationships, for it will reinforce, not detract from, the clarity of the role of each discipline.

If reorganising nursing care falls into the trap set by politicians and managers, there must indeed be caution in developing primary nursing. However, as has been suggested throughout this text, primary nursing is more than a mere restructuring of the hierarchy or a redeployment of actions and responsibilities. It is a whole new way of thinking about and carrying out nursing. To see it merely as reorganisation is to underestimate and misunderstand it.

To attempt to interpret and evaluate it in strict scientific terms also has its limitations. Professional judgment can be dismissed as subjective and therefore invalid. The living, qualitative relationship that can exist between nurse and patient can be dismissed as mere emotion, untranslatable into cost-effective terms. If primary nursing is in part a philosophy of care:

'then we must proceed with philosophic inquiry into the nature of primary nursing. In the absence of this inquiry, attempts at measuring the effects of primary nursing using scientific means are premature, for they will be as ineffective in the future as they have been in the past. Philosophic questions are not answerable through the scientific method. Whatever the source is of these problems, they must be addressed. To ignore them is to assume that research in nursing will not provide a sound basis for making decisions about ways and means of improving nursing care' (Giovanetti, 1987).

POWER AND PROFESSIONALISM IN PRIMARY NURSING

Many writers, such as Bowers (1989), seem to suggest that primary nursing is a symptom of professionalisation in nursing. It is a sign of the desire to become more powerful by being a profession. On this issue it is right to be cautious. If primary nursing encourages development of an élitist power group of nursing, all that will have happened is for power over patients to be transferred from one power group to another. Will nursing then fall into this traditional mould of professionalism, or is there an alternative for a nursing profession based on different values – the values inherent in primary nursing?

The difference here is a fundamentally important one, and it is an issue to which nurses in practice must address themselves in the onward rush to professional status. Should nursing be a profession? Nursing exists to serve the health needs of clients and patients. How can it organise itself so that the service position to the consumer is ensured, so that high standards of practice are maintained and developed? How can the construction of a monstrous professional megalith be avoided, which may in the end expend more energy in preserving its own integrity and value than in acting as the guardian of and supplicant to the patient's rights?

The interests of nurses and the interests of patients are one and the same, and both should be allies in the fight to resist the interests of the powerful few, especially in a time of increasingly élitist medicine and shrinking resources. Often dazzled by the white heat of the advance of medical technology and the power and prestige of medicine, the consumer's opportunity to exercise power and control over his own health needs are minimised. Nurses are befuddled by confused gender hierarchies (male/doctor dominance, female/nurse subservience) and trapped by the altruism of their calling. If only Florence Nightingale had trained her nurses in assertiveness instead of military obedience to dogma and authority! Miller (1979) argues that altruism has created a paradox for nursing. It may serve society but it does little to help the nurse. In addition, the nurses' subservient role hinders them in their fight as advocate of the patients' rights, when the patients themselves may not have the power to fight for themselves. Oakley (1984) notes that people who belong to subordinate groups such as nurses and women 'tend to be socialised into a psychological pattern which emphasises dependency, passivity, subservience, and thinking about other people's welfare'. The socially dominant groups, e.g. men or doctors, learn qualities of independence, initiative, control, domination and putting their own welfare and development ahead of other people. The issues involved are highly complex, and this book has already begun to address itself to some of them in examining the way in which nurses organise themselves, their rôle in the process of change and their relationships with other health workers.

Nurses in the practice of primary nursing must be in the vanguard of questioning the application of professionalism to nursing. A powerful élite commanding high status and salary would have to be smaller than at present; significant rises in pay could not be given to what is currently a massive, homogeneous group. Would this mean an even smaller body of trained nurses governing the activities of the untrained? Or might a system develop where the label 'professional' is only applied to relatively few nurses who have spent a longer period in vocational training (as doctors do)? Contrast this with the current system, which trains a nurse for 3 years, then considers her capable of full nursing responsibilities.

An awareness is developing among nurses of the value of nursing and of advancing their practice, not merely as a reflection of the narcissistic mirror that medicine offers, but in the mirror offered by the patient based on his level of satisfaction. The advanced 'professional nurse' is both teacher and healer, enhancing her own skills and knowledge, but in so doing offering these to patients so that they are in control of their own health and not subject to a market dominance or monopoly by nurses.

A fundamental philosophical shift of emphasis is required, which must be largely the task of nurses in practice. 'Power' to many nurses is almost a dirty word, but they must take it to act both on a political and personal level to serve their clients. Nursing must be a new kind of powerful profession, sharing, not hiding, knowledge and skill – open and working with clients as partners, not closed and controlling or dominating them. Having grasped power, nurses must then pass it right into the hands of patients, by working with them as partners or companions. Nurses would thus give a new character to the behaviour of a profession. Whatever form the changing face of nursing takes, however far it becomes 'professional', nurses in practice and those who support them must build the safeguards that ensure that nursing is the instrument of the patient, not the patient the instrument of nursing. This is one of the fundamental challenges of primary nursing.

CONCLUSION

There are many ways forward in nursing, and primary nursing is but one of them. It is a method of organising care based on certain essential philosophical assumptions about nursing. It is not just a means of redeploying the nursing team, but a whole way of thinking about nursing, which identifies it as valuable, creative, skilful and therapeutic in its own right. Primary nursing puts the trained nurse in a position to be accountable for, and autonomous in, giving the total nursing care of a patient or group of patients. The care is co-ordinated by that nurse, who may be assisted by others acting as his or her associate, in a comprehensive pattern throughout the patient's stay in his or her setting, and fully involves the patient, the family and other carers and members of the multidisciplinary team in the nursing of the patient.

To develop nursing in such a way may seem hopelessly unrealistic to many nurses. Beset by problems of resources and reorganisation, it is little wonder that primary nursing may be little more than a vision to many – a utopian dream that would be so nice, it's true – if only we had the staff, or supportive managers, or decent facilities!

The journey on the road towards primary nursing is fraught with difficulties. It needs complex and long-term plans to overcome them. Should we wait for research before we proceed? After all, primary nursing is not *proven* to be effective, and wouldn't it be safer just to stay as we are? Primary nurses and those who support them must be voyagers, for they venture out, often into uncharted territory it is true. If we always waited for evidence, for research, for clear maps to guide the way, we would never go anywhere. We would be afraid to turn the next corner for fear of the uncertainty that lies beyond it. This book has been an attempt to chart the territory of primary nursing a little more clearly.

The hopes in primary nursing may be branded as unrealistic. Those who promote it may be accused of not living in the 'real world'. Where primary nursing has succeeded, it has often been against considerable odds. Those nurses have not lived in an unreal world; they have simply set about creating a new reality for themselves, however long – sometimes years – it has taken.

The status quo does not seem to be an option. The Department of Health's nursing section (1989) has endorsed primary nursing as a way forward, recognising that there remain in nursing many dark corners of inadequate care (Martin, 1984; Health Service Ombudsman, 1986, 1987, 1988). New initiatives are needed to improve standards of care. Encouragement from these and other quarters (or from managers who might see it as a means to greater control in cost-cutting) needs to be treated with caution. Otherwise there is a risk that this support transforms into a rod with which to beat the clinical nurses (you *must* do primary nursing because the Department says so!!). Primary nursing needs extensive preparation, continued support and time, perhaps many years, to grow.

All nursing before primary nursing was not bad, and all that follows it will not inevitably be good. Primary nursing is not a panacea. It will not cure nursing's ills overnight. It will not suddenly produce patients who are loving and co-operative, it will not instantly remove interdisciplinary conflicts and it will not make nurses immediately kind to one another. All nurses will not suddenly become expert communicators, night staff will not quickly lose their sense of isolation and nurses will not cease to go 'off sick'. What primary nursing will do is enable nurses to confront these and many more issues of conflict in nursing and, more importantly, empower them to do something about it. Primary nursing may produce conflicts, but many of them are problems we have long covered up. Tackling them is long overdue.

Primary nursing will only work where nurses are ready and willing to take on board their accountability and autonomy, to work with colleagues in a relationship of equals, and to share care with patients and other carers as partners and companions. It will only work when managers and educators take on their rightful role as supporters of clinical nursing, not just its controllers. The more you control, the less you create.

If success does not come as fast as we would wish, it is right to remember that it is not all our fault! If you are not instantly achieving in primary nursing, it may not be your problem, so do not feel guilty. Nurses often take the guilt of their failings onto their own shoulders. It should be remembered that others play a part too – those who are unhelpful or obstructive. In this case, when guilty feelings arrive, perhaps it is worthwhile off-loading them to the real source of the problem.

Meanwhile, value and cherish what you do that makes care personal. There is much that can be done to make life better for patients that does not depend on primary nursing.

Primary nursing is part of a long process of change in nursing, in which nursing and its inherent values are reawakened and its territory rediscovered and redefined. If nurses do not do this, others will – and not necessarily to the benefit of patients. Primary nursing is a way of thinking and working with patients that challenges established practices and undermines outmoded customs. Nurses in primary nursing are the termites of the nursing establishment. However, all this must be for the practical benefit of patients, otherwise it is mere intellectual tennis. It is the challenge to nursing to work with patients as people, test out our values and redefine our practice.

It is the call for the nurse to work with 'my patients', to provide the humane personal help and healing which the patients want from 'my nurse'. Pursue your vision!

APPENDIX

Sample Job Descriptions for Primary Nursing

Please note that these are examples of job descriptions only. Modifications will need to be made for permanent night duty staff, where the night nurse is likely to be an associate nurse yet carry additional supervisory, clinical and managerial responsibilities [e.g. night nurses (associate) are graded on scales from D through to F to reflect these factors].

JOB DESCRIPTION 1

Role: Care assistant

Grade: A

Responsible to: Deputy UGM/head of nursing services (Unit I) through the senior nurse manager (Care of the Elderly and Nursing Development Unit)

Accountable to: Senior primary nurse/primary nurse

Job summary:
The principal aim of the care assistant's role is to support the primary nurse/associate nurse in the delivery of nursing care. This may be by directly assisting the nurse with his/her caseload of patients or by helping with general ward organisation.
The post-holder will:

- Assist the primary/associate nurse as required in the giving of care, within the unit's agreed guidelines for the activities of the care assistant.
- Assist with general orderliness of the ward.
- Carry out delegated non-nursing activities to assist the primary nurse/associate nurse.
- Assist with appropriate aspects of nursing care under supervision.
- Contribute to maintaining the ward's agreed philosophy, aims and objectives.
- Keep the primary/associate nurse informed of observations relating to patient care.
- Work with colleagues to help co-ordinate nursing and other activities on the ward.
- Follow agreed unit and health authority policies in relation to personal and patient safety.
- Keep up to date by attending to personal development, attending appropriate lectures, etc.
- Maintain the confidentiality of the patients and their care.
- Work as part of the team to promote a climate on the ward conducive to learning and high standards of patient care.

This job description is intended to give a broad outline to the function and responsibilities of the care assistant and may be updated at regular intervals.

A job description is not a rigid or inflexible document but acts to provide guidelines to the duties expected while in post.

This job description will be reviewed and amended in the light of changing professional demands.

JOB DESCRIPTION 2

Role: Associate nurse

Grade: C

Responsible to: Deputy UGM/head of nursing services

(Unit I) through the senior nurse manager (Care of the Elderly and Nursing Development Unit)

Accountable to: Senior primary nurse/primary nurse

Minimum qualifications: State enrolled nurse

Job profile:

The associate nurse works under the direction of the primary nurse to assess, plan, implement and evaluate the nursing care of a given caseload of patients.

The post-holder will:

Clinical

- Give care to patients under the direction of the primary nurse.
- Assist with the assessing, planning, implementing and evaluation of care.
- Liaise with the primary nurse to co-ordinate the overall plan of care.
- Accurately document nursing care.
- Work according to the ward's agreed philosophy, nursing model and objectives.
- Work with the primary nurse to produce a therapeutic ward environment for patient care.

Educational

- Keep up to date with current nursing practice.
- Accept responsibility for maintaining professional development and identify own learning needs.
- Help colleagues by passing on expertise to others and participate in the overall plans of the ward to promote learning.

Management

- Assist in the supervision of care assistants.
- Co-ordinate his or her own activities with the rest of the ward to ensure achievements of the ward's objectives.

- Work according to unit and health authority policies and the UKCC Code of Conduct.
- Promote the safety of self, colleagues and patients at all times, in relation to equipment, the ward environment, etc.
- Take part in other duties as agreed within the unit's policies.

Research

- Make use of appropriate research findings in nursing practice.
- Co-operate with colleagues with research projects and the evaluation of care.

A job description is not a rigid or inflexible document but acts to provide guidelines to the duties expected while in post.

This job description will be reviewed and amended in the light of changing professional demands.

JOB DESCRIPTION 3

Role: Associate nurse

Scale: D

Responsible to: Deputy UGM/head of nursing services (Unit I) through the senior nurse manager (Care of the Elderly and Nursing Development Unit)

Accountable to: Primary nurse/senior primary nurse

Minimum qualifications: RGN/SEN with relevant post-qualification experience

Job profile:
1. The post-holder is responsible for assisting with the assessment of care needs and the development of programmes of care, and/or the implementation and evaluation of these programmes.
2. The post-holder is expected to carry out all relevant forms of care without direct supervision and may be required to

demonstrate procedures to, and supervise, qualified and/
or unqualified staff.
The post-holder will:

Clinical

- Be a safe practitioner.
- Liaise with and provide relevant information to other
members of the multiprofessional team.
- Assist in the facilitating of a therapeutic environment
that meets the needs of the patients.
- Take responsibility for a caseload of patients in the
absence of the primary nurse.
- Co-ordinate the patient's care with the primary nurse.
- Assess, plan, implement, evaluate and document care in
association with the primary nurse.
- Work with colleagues to promote the development of the
ward's philosophy, nursing model and agreed clinical
objectives.
- Work with colleagues to develop clinical expertise and
high standards of nursing practice.

Research

- Demonstrate a commitment to developing his or her own
research skills.
- Be receptive and supportive towards the research plans
of others.
- Contribute to the application and evaluation of current
research findings.

Management

- Occasionally take responsibility for the management of
the ward and patient care in the absence of a more senior
nurse.
- In the absence of a more senior nurse, be responsible for
the co-ordination of all activities within the ward.
- Help to maintain positive working relationships with the
multidisciplinary team.

- Ensure the promotion of safety, well-being and interests of patients, staff and all visitors to the clinical area.
- Be aware of the district health authority policies and procedures and carry these out in the clinical area.
- At all times follow the Code of Professional Conduct as laid down by the UKCC.

Educational

- Under the guidance of senior sister/charge nurse (scale G), identify own learning needs.
- Assist in the facilitating of a learning environment conducive to the acquisition of further knowledge and skills.
- Contribute, where appropriate, to the development of teaching strategies, taking into account the needs of staff and patients.
- Liaise with colleagues to co-ordinate the approach to the development of staff in the ward.

A job description is not a rigid or inflexible document but acts to provide guidelines to the duties expected while in post.

This job description will be reviewed and amended in the light of changing professional demands.

JOB DESCRIPTION 4

Role: Primary nurse

Scale: E

Responsible to: Deputy UGM/head of nursing services (Unit I) through the senior nurse manager (Care of the Elderly and Nursing Development Unit)

Accountable to: Senior primary nurse/senior sister/charge nurse (scale G)

Minimum qualifications: RGN plus at least 6 months post-registration experience and evidence of further development in the speciality with particular reference to preparation for primary nursing.

Job profile:
1. The post-holder is responsible for the assessment of care needs and the development, implementation and evaluation of programmes of care.
2. The post-holder is expected to carry out all relevant forms of care and may take charge regularly of a ward or equivalent sphere of nursing in the absence of the person who has continuing responsibility. The post-holder is expected to supervise junior staff and will be expected to teach qualified and unqualified staff, including basic and/or post-basic students, where applicable.
3. The post-holder is required to take responsibility as the primary nurse for a defined group of patients and may act as an associate nurse in the absence of a colleague. He/she works with minimal supervision in the assessment of all relevant care needs and in the development, implementation and evaluation of programmes of care.
4. The post-holder is expected to participate fully in quality assurance initiatives, with particular emphasis on a 'customer first' approach.

The post-holder will:

Management

- Take responsibility for the management of the ward and patient care in the absence of a more senior nurse, with the aim of setting the highest possible standards.
- In the absence of a more senior nurse, be responsible for the co-ordination of all activities within the ward or equivalent sphere.
- Help to create and maintain positive working relationships within the multidisciplinary team.
- Ensure the promotion of safety, well-being and interests of the patients, staff and all visitors to the clinical area.
- Be aware of the district health authority policies and procedures and carry these out in the clinical areas, and ensure that all junior staff follow these policies and procedures.
- At all times follow the Code of Professional Conduct as laid down by the UKCC and ensure that all staff within

this sphere of responsibility also follow the code as laid down.
- Contribute to monitoring the performance of staff within the sphere of responsibility and report to the senior sister/charge nurse (scale G).

Clinical

- Demonstrate clinical excellence.
- Liaise with, and provide relevant information to, other members of the multiprofessional team.
- Assist in the supervision and monitoring of nursing practice under the guidance of the senior sister/charge nurse (scale G).
- Assist in the facilitating of a therapeutic environment that meets the needs of the patients.
- Carry a clinical caseload as a primary nurse, and act as an associate nurse for colleagues where appropriate.
- Contribute to the development of the ward's philosophy and nursing model.
- Contribute to meeting the agreed clinical objectives for the ward.
- Work with senior colleagues to develop further clinical expertise and develop soundly based nursing practice.

Research

- Demonstrate commitment to developing their own research skills.
- Be receptive and supportive towards the research plans of others.
- Contribute to the application and evaluation of current research into care.
- Participate in appropriate research/evaluation studies on the ward.
- Contribute to the documentation of the activities of the ward.

Educational

- Contribute as a counsellor and adviser to the learners and other ward staff on matters related to care of the elderly in the absence of a more senior nurse.
- Accept personal responsibility for identifying his or her own learning needs and professional development.
- Assist in the facilitating of a learning environment conducive to the acquisition of further knowledge and skills.
- Contribute to the development of teaching strategies appropriate to the needs of staff and patients.
- Be prepared to accept the role of a preceptor/mentor.
- Liaise with all colleagues in a teaching capacity to ensure an overall co-ordinated approach to staff development.

A job description is not a rigid or inflexible document but acts to provide guidelines to the duties expected while in post.

This job description will be reviewed and amended in the light of changing professional demands.

JOB DESCRIPTION 5

Role: Primary nurse/sister/charge nurse
Scale: F
Responsible to: Deputy UGM/head of nursing services (Unit I) through the senior nurse manager (Care of the Elderly and Nursing Development Unit)
Accountable to: Senior primary nurse/sister/charge nurse (continuing responsibility – scale G)
Minimum qualifications: RGN plus at least 2 years appropriate post-registration experience including evidence of further development in the speciality.
Job profile:
1. The post-holder is designated to take charge regularly of a clinical area of nursing in the absence of the person who has continuing responsibility.

2. The post-holder is responsible for the assessment of care needs and the development, implementation and evaluation of programmes of care, without supervision, and may be required to teach other nursing and non-nursing staff.

3. The post-holder will be a primary nurse who may also act as an associate nurse for colleagues.

4. The post-holder will be required to act up for the G grade.

5. The post-holder is expected to participate fully in quality assurance initiatives with particular emphasis on a 'customer first' approach.

The post-holder will:

Managerial

- Take responsibility for the management of the clinical area in the absence of the sister/charge nurse (scale G), with the aim of setting the highest possible standards, following the agreed guidelines laid down in the ward's philosophy of care/aims and objectives.
- Help to create and maintain positive relationships between all groups involved in the welfare of the patient.
- Be responsible for the co-ordination of all activities in the absence of the sister/charge nurse (scale G).
- Ensure the promotion of safety, well-being and interests of the patients, staff and visitors to the clinical area.
- Communicate as necessary to all staff the district health authority policies and procedures and carry these out in the clinical areas, and inform all junior staff of any changes to them so that they follow these policies and procedures.
- At all times follow the Code of Professional Conduct as laid down by the UKCC and ensure that all staff within their sphere of responsibility also follow the code as laid down.
- Assist and support the sister/charge nurse (scale G) in planning staff duty rotas to meet the requirements of the unit and clinical areas.
- Monitor the performance of staff within their sphere of

responsibility and report to the sister/charge nurse (scale G).

Clinical

- Demonstrate clinical expertise and act as a positive role model.
- Act as a clinical adviser to the multiprofessional team.
- Be responsible for supervising and monitoring nursing practice under the guidance of the sister/charge nurse (scale G).
- Facilitate a therapeutic environment that meets the needs of the patients.
- Contribute to the development of the ward's philosophy and nursing model to promote the aims of personal nursing care.
- Act as a primary nurse and co-ordinate the care of a given caseload of patients from admission through to discharge.
- Participate in pursuing the agreed ward objectives in the promotion of high standards of care.
- Strive to ensure that all nursing practice is based on sound rationale.
- Accurately pursue and document the assessment, planning, implementation and evaluation of nursing care.

Research

- Demonstrate a commitment to developing research skills in themselves and junior staff.
- Be receptive to the research plans of others and encourage full co-operation with all the staff.
- Assist in the application and evaluation of current research findings.
- Participate in appropriate research/evaluation studies on the ward.
- Contribute to the documentation of activities/evaluation of care on the ward.

Educational

- Participate in the teaching and development of all grades of staff on the ward.
- Act as mentor/preceptor where appropriate.
- Identify own learning/development needs and take steps to pursue objectives.
- Liaise with the senior primary nurse/ward sister/charge nurse to co-ordinate teaching/learning activities on the ward.
- Contribute as a counsellor and adviser to the learners and other staff on matters related to the care of the elderly.
- Facilitate a learning environment conducive to the acquisition of further knowledge and skills.

This job description is not a rigid or inflexible document but acts to provide guidelines to the duties expected while in post.

This job description will be reviewed and amended in the light of changing professional demands.

JOB DESCRIPTION 6

Role: Senior primary nurse/sister/charge nurse (continuing responsibility)

Scale: G

Responsible to: Deputy UGM/head of nursing services (Unit I)

Accountable to: Senior nurse manager (Care of the Elderly and Nursing Development Unit)

Minimum qualifications: RGN with appropriate post-registration experience, including evidence of further development in the fields of teaching, primary nursing, management, care of the elderly and research.

Job profile:
The post holder:

1. Carries continuing responsibility over a 24-hour period

for the assessment of care needs, the development, implementation and evaluation of programmes of care and the setting of standards of care.
2. Carries continuing responsibility for the management of a clinical area of nursing (one ward), including the deployment and supervision of staff, the teaching of all staff and/or learners and the provision of advice within the clinical area.
3. Carries specific multiprofessional co-ordinating responsibilities over the 24-hour period.
4. Will be the designated budget holder.
5. Will act up for the senior nurse manager in her absence.
6. Will participate in and encourage all quality assurance initiatives with particular emphasis on a 'customer first' approach.
7. Will liaise with the consultant nurse and clinical nurse specialists as appropriate.
8. Will annually identify written personal objectives with the senior nurse manager, head of nursing services and consultant nurse.

By working individually and with colleagues the postholder will:

Management

- Be responsible for the continuous management of the clinical area of nursing over 24 hours, with the aim of setting the highest possible standards, following the agreed unit philosophy.
- Be responsible for budgetary control for their clinical area of nursing.
- Be responsible for the creation and maintenance of positive working relationships within the multidisciplinary team.
- Be responsible for the co-ordination of all activities within the clinical area of nursing.
- – Ensure the promotion of safety, well-being and interests of the patients, staff and all visitors to the clinical area.

– Pay particular regard to the district health authority's fire procedures.

- Act as change agent to promote innovation and high standard of practice.
- Communicate to all staff the district's policies and procedures, inform all staff of any changes to them and ensure that staff follow these policies and procedures.
- Inform the representatives of each committee, should procedures or policies require updating.
- At all times follow the Code of Professional Conduct as laid down by the UKCC and ensure that all staff within their sphere of responsibility also follow the code as laid down.
- Plan the staff duty rotas to meet the requirements of the unit, ward and patients' needs and to facilitate primary nursing.
- Monitor and appraise the performance of staff within their sphere of responsibility.
- Monitor nurse–patient dependency levels.
- Monitor staff sickness and absence and take appropriate managerial action.
- Work on day and night duty shifts as appropriate to meet the needs of 24-hour responsibility for the ward.

Clinical

- Demonstrate clinical excellence and high standards of nursing practice to other staff.
- Be responsible for supervising and monitoring nursing practice and be accountable for the same.
- Develop a therapeutic environment that meets the needs of the patients.
- Work with colleagues to set standards of clinical nursing and organise care to achieve these.
- Retain a clinical input by acting as a primary or associate nurse.
- Promote clinical activities that give appropriate partici- pation to patients, relatives and other carers in the process of care.

- Meet clinical objectives as agreed separately with the senior nurse manager and consultant nurse.
- Identify and develop a model of nursing practice to promote the goals of personal nursing care.
- Ensure that the care of all patients is assessed, planned, implemented, evaluated and appropriately documented.

Research

- Demonstrate a commitment to developing research skills in themselves and other staff.
- Be receptive to the research plans of others and encourage full co-operation from all staff.
- Apply, where appropriate, and evaluate findings of current research into patient care.
- Carry out studies and research projects appropriate to the field of expertise.
- Identify areas of study/research on the ward, document these activities and review with the consultant nurse for wider dissemination of findings/activities.
- Develop methods at ward level to monitor standards of care in liaison with the clinical nurse specialist (quality assurance/research).

Educational

- Act as a counsellor and adviser to students and other ward staff related to care of the elderly.
- Accept personal responsibility for identifying own learning needs and professional development.
- Develop a learning environment conducive to the acquisition of further knowledge for all staff.
- Identify the training needs of all staff within their sphere of responsibility and develop teaching strategies appropriate to the needs of staff and patients.
- Be an ENB assessor.
- Accept the role of preceptor where applicable.
- Act as a role model and mentor to colleagues in the demonstration of high standards of practice.
- Liaise with other staff involved in education in the unit

to provide a cohesive approach to the development of students and staff.

- Act as a clinical adviser to the multiprofessional team.

A job description is not a rigid or inflexible document but acts to provide guidelines to the duties expected while in post.

This job description will be reviewed and amended in the light of changing professional demands.

References

Argyle M. (1978) *The Psychology of Interpersonal Behaviour.* Harmondsworth: Penguin.

Aschjem O., Carlsen L.B. and Markussen A.B. (1979) Primaersykepleie lever i norge, og har det ganske bra! *Sykepleien,* **66**(17): 6–11, 13.

Benner P. (1984) *From Novice to Expert.* London: Addison Wesley.

Bergman R. (1981) Accountability – definition and dimensions. *International Nursing Review,* **28**(2): 53–59.

Beyers M. and Phillips C. (1971) *Nursing Management for Patient Care.* Boston: Little, Brown.

Binnie A. (1987) Primary nursing: structural changes. *Nursing Times,* **83**(39): 36–37.

Blanpain J.E. (1976) Systems analysis of the nursing unit: primary nursing, a holistic approach to the delivery of nursing care. Unpublished document cited in *The Change to Primary Nursing* (1982) Hegyvary S.T. London: C. V. Mosby.

Bowers L. (1989) The significance of primary nursing. *Journal of Advanced Nursing,* **14**: 13–19.

Campbell A.V. (1984) *Moderated Love.* London: SPCK.

Dean D. (1988) *Manpower Solutions.* London: RCN.

Department of Health (1989) *A Strategy for Nursing.* London: DoH.

Dimond B. (1988) *The Law and the Nurse.* Unpublished paper, Nursing Times Primary Nursing Conference, Manchester.

English National Board for Nursing, Midwifery and Health Visiting (1987a) *Circular No. MAT/28.* London: ENB.

English National Board for Nursing, Midwifery and Health Visiting (1987b) *Managing Change in Nursing Education.* London: ENB.

Georgiades N.J. and Phillimore L. (1975) The myth of the hero-innovator. In: *Behaviour Modification with the Severely Retarded,* eds. Kiernan C.C. and Woodford F.P. London: ASP.

Giovanetti P. (1987) Evaluation of primary nursing. *Annual Review of Nursing Research,* **1**(4): 127–151.

Hall L.E. (1969) The Loeb Centre for Nursing and Rehabilitation. *International Journal of Nursing Studies*, **6:** 82–83.

Health Service Ombudsman (1986, 1987, 1988) *Reports of the Health Service Parliamentary Liaison Officer (Ombudsman)*. London: DHSS.

Hegyvary S.T. (1982) *The Change to Primary Nursing*. London: C.V. Mosby.

Henderson V. (1980) Preserving the essence of nursing in a technological age. *Journal of Advanced Nursing*, **5:** 245–260.

Kafka F. (1916) *Metamorphosis* (reprinted 1974). Harmondsworth: Penguin.

Kramer M. (1974) *Reality Shock*. St Louis: C.V. Mosby.

Lanara V. (1981) *Heroism as a Nursing Value*. Athens: Sisterhood Evniki.

Lathlean J. (1988) Viable reality or pipe dream? *Nursing Times*, **84**(49): 39–40.

Lee M.E. (1979) Towards better care: primary nursing. *Nursing Times* occasional paper, **75**(33): 133–135.

MacDonald M. (1988) Primary nursing: is it worth it? *Journal of Advanced Nursing*, **13:** 797–806.

MacGuire J. (1988) Does mix matter? In: *Options and Opportunities*, DHSS. London: DHSS.

Machiavelli N. (1514) *The Prince* (translation by G. Bull, reprinted 1986). Harmondsworth: Penguin.

Manthey M. (1970) Primary nursing. *Nursing Forum*, **IX**(1): 65–83.

Manthey M. (1973) Primary nursing is alive and well in the hospital. *American Journal of Nursing*, **73:** 83–87.

Manthey M. (1980) *The Practice of Primary Nursing*. London: Blackwell.

Manthey M. (1988) Can primary nursing survive? *American Journal of Nursing*, **88:** 644–647.

Marks-Maran D. (1978) Patient allocation v task allocation in relation to the nursing process. *Nursing Times*, **74**(10): 413–416.

Marram G.D. (1976) The comparative costs of operating team or primary nursing. *Journal of Nursing Administration*, **6**(4): 21–24.

Martin J.P. (1984) *Hospitals in Trouble*. London: Blackwell.

McFarlane J. and Castledine G. (1982) *A Guide to the Practice of Nursing Using the Nursing Process*. London: C. V. Mosby.

McLure M.L., Poulin M.A., Sovie M.D. and Wandelt M.A. (1983) *Magnet Hospitals – Attraction and Retention of Professional Nurses*. Kansas City: American Academy of Nursing.

Medaglia M. (1978) A coronary care unit implements primary nursing. *Canadian Nurse*, **74**(5): 32–34.

Menzies I. (1961) The functioning of social systems as a defence against anxiety (reprinted 1988). In: *Containing Anxiety in Institutions*, Menzies-Lyth I. (1988). London: Free Associate Books.

Miller J.B. (1979) *Towards a new Psychology of Women*. Boston: Beacon Press.

Nightingale F. (1869) *Notes on Nursing, What It Is and What It Is Not* (republished 1980). Edinburgh: Churchill Livingstone.

Oakley A. (1984) The importance of being a nurse. *Nursing Times*, **80**(50): 24–27.

Otoya T. (1979) Advantages and disadvantages of team nursing: a trial at primary nursing. *Kangogaku Zasshi*, **43**: 163–169.

Ottoway R.N. (1976) A change strategy to implement new norms, new styles and new environment in the work organisation. *Personnel Review*, **5**(1): 13–18.

Ottoway R.N. (1980) *Defining the Change Agent*. Unpublished Research Paper. Department of Management Sciences, University of Manchester Institute of Technology.

Pearson A. (1985) *The Effects of Introducing New Norms in a Nursing Unit; An Analysis of the Process of Change*. Unpublished PhD thesis, Goldsmith College, University of London.

Pearson A. (ed.) (1988a) *Primary Nursing*. London: Croom Helm.

Pearson A. (1988b) Trends in clinical nursing. In: *Primary Nursing*, ed. Pearson A. London: Croom Helm.

Pearson A. and Vaughan B. (1986) *Nursing Models for Practice*. London: Heinemann.

Pembrey S. (1980) *The Ward Sister – Key to Nursing*. London: RCN.

Price Waterhouse (1988) *Nurse Retention and Recruitment*. London: Price Waterhouse.

Purdy E., Wright S.G. and Johnson M.L. (1988) Change for the better. *Nursing Times*, **84**(38): 34–36.

RCN (1986) *The Education of Nurses: A New Dispensation*. London: RCN.

Reilly D. (1975) Why a conceptual framework? *Nursing Outlook*, **23**(9): 12–20.

Remington I. (1989) Night rites. *Nursing Times*, **85**(1): 30–31.

Rotkontch R. (1979) Personal communication. Cited in *The Change to Primary Nursing* (1982), Hegyvary S.T. London: C.V. Mosby.

Salvage J. (1985) *The Politics of Nursing*. London: Heinemann.

Salvage J. (1988) *Facilitating Model Based Nursing*. Unpublished paper. Nursing Models Conference, Gateshead.

Shukla R.K. (1983) An all RN model of nursing care delivery; a cost benefit evaluation. *Inquiry*, **20**: 173–184.

Sparrow S. (1986) Primary nursing. *Nursing Practice*, 1(3): 142–147.

Stein L. (1978) The doctor–nurse game. In: *Readings in the Sociology of Nursing*, eds. Dingwall R. and MacIntosh J. Edinburgh: Churchill Livingstone.

Stockwell F. (1972) *The Unpopular Patient*. London: RCN.

Strong P. and Robinson J. (1988) *New Model Management: Griffiths and the NHS*. Warwick: Nursing Policy Studies Centre, University of Warwick.

Turrill T. (1985) *Change and Innovation: A Challenge for the NHS*, Management Series 10. London: Institution of Health Service Management.

Tutton L. (1986) What is primary nursing? *Professional Nurse*, 2(2): 39–40.

United Kingdom Central Council for Nursing, Midwifery and Health Visiting (1983) *Code of Professional Conduct for the Nurse, Midwife and Health Visitor*. London: UKCC.

United Kingdom Central Council for Nursing, Midwifery and Health Visiting (1986) *Project 2000*. London: UKCC.

Van Eindhoven J.M.B. (1979) Patient-orientated ward organisation. *International Nursing Review*, 26: 3.

Waters K. (1985) Team nursing. *Nursing Practice*, 1(1): 7–15.

Watson J. (1978) Patient evaluation of primary nursing project. *Australian Nurses Journal*, 8(5): 30–33.

Wills G. (1988) An evaluation of primary nursing in a continuing care/rehabilitation ward. Unpublished survey, Nursing Development Unit, Tameside General Hospital.

Wills G. and Wright S.G. (1988) Getting to know you. *Nursing Standard*, 3(9): 32.

Woods D. (1987) *Biko*. Harmondsworth: Penguin.

Wright S.G. (1986) *Building and Using a Model of Nursing*. London: Arnold.

Wright S.G. (1987a) Consuming interests. *Senior Nurse*, 62: 24–26.

Wright S.G. (1987b) Patient centred practice. *Nursing Times*, 83(38): 24–29.

Wright S.G. (1988) The bandwagon effect. *Nursing Standard*, 3(5): 42.

Wright S.G. (1989) *Changing Nursing Practice*. London: Edward Arnold.

Wright S.G. and Purdy E. (1988) If I were a rich nurse. *Nursing Times*, 84(41): 36–37.

Young J.P., Giovanetti P., Lewison D. and Thomas M.L. (1981) *Factors Affecting Nurse Staffing in Acute Care Hospitals; A Review and Critique of the Literature* (DHEW Publication no. HRP050180C). Hyattsville, USA: Department of Health Education and Welfare.

Index